Ra5,
good luck. We're gonna
miss you. I hope that
This book will remind you
of me when I'm not
around.

Eric S. Rabkin
Eugene M. Silverman

IT'S A GAS

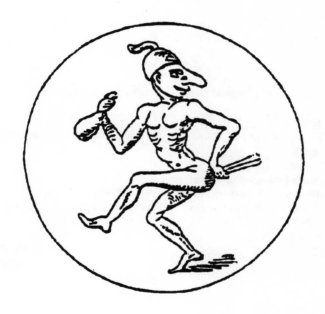

A Study of Flatulence

XENOS BOOKS

Copyright © 1991
by Eric S. Rabkin & Eugene M. Silverman

All rights reserved.

Library of Congress Cataloging-in-Publication Data

Rabkin, Eric S.
  It's a gas : a study of flatulence / by Eric S. Rabkin and Eugene
M. Silverman.
    p.   cm.
  Includes bibliographical references.
  ISBN 1-879378-04-3 (cloth) -- ISBN 1-879378-03-5 (pbk)
    1. Flatulence--Popular works.   I. Silverman, Eugene M. (Eugene
Morton), 1938-   .   II. Title.
RC862.F55R33   1991
612.3--dc20   91-26010
                                                             CIP
                                                              r91

Designed by Karl Kvitko. Published by Xenos Books, P.O.
Box 52152, Riverside, CA. 92517-3152. Printed in the United
States of America by Van Volumes Ltd., Thorndike, MA. 01079.

ACKNOWLEDGMENTS

"The Miller's Tale" from *The Portable Chaucer* edited and translated by Theodore Morrison. Copyright 1949 by Theodore Morrison. Copyright renewed 1976 by Theodore Morrison. Reprinted by permission of Viking Penguin Inc.

"The Historic Fart" from *Tales from the Thousand & One Nights*, trans. N. J. Dawood (Penguin Classics, Revised edition 1973), pp. 163-164. Translation copyright © N.J. Dawood, 1954, 1973. Reprinted by permission of Penguin Books Ltd.

Excerpt from *La Terre*, Emile Zola, translated by Ann Lindsay, copyright 1954. Reprinted by permission of Granada Publishing Limited.

"Lysistrata Defending the Acropolis," Aubrey Beardsley, taken from *The Collected Drawings of Aubrey Beardsley*. Copyright © 1978 by Crown Publishers, Inc. Used by permission of Crown Publishers, Inc.

*This book is
respectfully dedicated
to
Messrs.
Stokeley, Heinz and Van Camp*

For Freedom of Expression
— or, what's wrong with fart? —

> *What comfort can the vortices*
> *of Descartes give to a man who*
> *has whirlwinds in his bowels!*

Benjamin Franklin

We all do it, but we can't talk about it. And why not? In some cultures people pass a happy afternoon in contesting who can pass the most gas, but in our culture we don't even have a simple, acceptable word for it. How can you find a place in ordinary conversation for words like flatulation, eructation, emanation or crepitation? Yet on the other hand what polite person would insult decent ears with phrases like let one fly, cut the cheese, break wind or blow off? What's wrong with fart? Why the secrecy? They put peppermints by restaurant exits, but they don't tell you why. We have been the victims of censorship too long! Did *you* know that a nineteenth century Frenchman made his living by farting music in night clubs? that a woman from Madison, Wisconsin exploded when an electric current ignited her flatus? that the word fart comes from the same root as the word partridge, the very bird that's been messing up your pear tree? Did you know *why* beans make you fart? Did you know that nearly 10 percent of the population have chronic excessive flatulence for bona fide medical reasons and that these people can be helped by simply changing their diet?

Every one of these facts is true. Holding back like this stinks to high heaven. There's Freedom of the Press to be considered — and the public's Right to Know. So in this book we blow the lid off. From the latest medical information to the suppressed works of literary masters, from true case histories to fanciful drawings, this book lets it all out of the bag. Once and for all, it's time to clear the air!

ESR
EMS

CONTENTS

it's a gas...

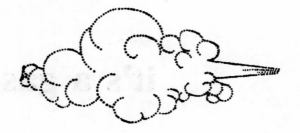

CHAPTER ONE

What's in a Fart?

— a medical dialogue —

> It is best for flatulence to pass without
> noise and breaking, though it is better
> for it to pass with noise than to be in-
> tercepted and accumulated internally.

Hippocrates, c. 420 B.C.

— Take me to Kennedy Airport.

— Okay, but that'll take a while with this traffic.

— Do the best you can, will you? I've got to catch a plane.

— No kiddin'? I thought you had to catch a boat.

— Look, are you gonna drive or just fart around?

— Oh, hey, I hadn't noticed. I mean, that was just a figure of speech.

— Yeah, I know.

— Look, I'm sorry. I've got this problem and I'll keep the air conditioner on.

— In November?

— It's for you, not me.

— Have you thought of seeing a doctor about this?

— Sure. Man, I live on tips. But the doctors just tell me to quit swallowing air.

— Aerophagia is an occasional cause of flatulence.

— Are you a doc?

1

— As a matter of fact, I am. I specialize in exactly your area of concern.

— Gas?

— Well, that depends on what you mean. Abdominal pain, distention of the stomach, excessive belching, abnormal flatulation, they're all my camp. But lots of other things that people call gas aren't. Air swallowing is a maybe.

— Well, am I swallowing air?

— I don't know, but you can find out easily enough. Just look in a mirror while you're having a chat. When you swallow, your Adam's apple, the larynx, moves up and down. If you see that happening while the *other* guy is talking and you're not eating, drinking or smoking, then you're swallowing air.

— Is that bad?

— No, but it can be uncomfortable, and if you keep eating garlic it might offend your passengers.

— Sorry, doc.

— Forget it. You can cure it anyway. It's hard, like breaking any other habit, but it can be done. Tie a string around your neck just over the larynx. Every time you swallow you'll feel it and that'll remind you not to do it. Until you do stop, you can relieve your passengers' problem by changing your diet; you can relieve your own problems by belching on purpose.

— You're kidding.

— No I'm not. And I should mention that sometimes aerophagia accompanies rapid eating, which can also be stopped if you just pay attention to it or force yourself to chew more slowly.

— But that can't be all there is to gas?

— No, aerophagia is just a simple functional problem. It only happens to be the most common one.

— What does "functional" mean?

— It means that all the parts are there and look normal, at least as far as we can tell, but that they may not be functioning properly.

— Is that possible?

— Sure. And sometimes it's easy to tell. If the discomfort comes only right after a big meal, you might well be suffering from "magenblase syndrome." This comes from a build-up of gas in the stomach during eating and may require a good belch.

— Urp.

— Very good. But if the discomfort doesn't come only right after a big meal and you still feel bloated there could be other causes.

— For example?

— Well, another functional difficulty is accumulation of gas in a flexure.

— Is that like a Lexus?

— Look, I'd better fill you in on some basics. When you swallow food, it goes down a tube called the esophagus and into the stomach. The stomach is closed at the bottom by a ring of muscle called the pylorus. From that ring begins the small intestine. Food gets digested in the stomach and small intestine, broken down into smaller chemical units that can be absorbed through the wall of the intestine into the bloodstream. The small intestine is a small diameter tube about twenty feet long all coiled up in your abdomen. The circular muscles of this tube keep the foodstuffs moving along by peristalsis, a motion kind of like squeezing a salami out of a salami skin with two hands.

— I thought that salami was out — too much garlic.

— Just don't turn off the air conditioner.

— Very funny.

— To continue, assuming you really want to learn about this material.

— I do, I do.

— All right then. The small intestine ends up way down in your abdomen and then, past another ring of muscle, opens up into a wide tube, the large intestine, that goes up toward the liver on your right, across your stomach to the spleen on the left and then back down until it finally ends up in the rectum.

— So what's a flexure?

— A flexure is a bend. The bend in the large intestine near the liver is the hepatic flexure. The bend near the spleen is the splenic flexure. Since the actual bend itself is a bit higher than the part of the large intestine that goes across, gas can get trapped in the flexures and cause pain.

— So what do you do about that?

— In some cases the patient finds relief simply by manipulating himself.

— Really? I thought that caused blindness.

— Not that kind of manipulation. What I had in mind was lying down with your knees to your chest and rocking back and forth. For many people a brisk walk or jog helps and for some, even hanging upside down.

— What?

— Yes. Just like sending a bubble through a tube of shampoo. But don't do it the very first time you feel a gas pain, in case the symptoms aren't reflecting trapped gas.

— What else could they reflect?

— Well, if the gas is trapped on the right, the pain in that region might be misdiagnosed as gall bladder problems. If that's the trouble, you don't lose anything by hanging off a

4

sturdy table. But if the bubble is on the left, the symptoms could be pain in the chest.

— Like a heart attack?

— Right. And if you are having a heart attack, it's usually not considered a good idea to hang upside down from anything.

— So what should you do?

— That's the time to turn the problem over to a doctor. And while you're waiting for the doctor, relax as much as you can. If it's a heart attack, relaxation will only help. And if it's gas in the splenic flexure, maybe the easing up of the muscles and the change of position will help you fart. In that case, breaking wind is definitely a good thing.

— And if it's a heart attack and no one helps you?

— You'll certainly begin to believe that gas is a minor problem.

— Who do you think you're making fun of, buddy?

— Excuse me. I can tell that this isn't really funny in your case.

— You're damned right. But look, where does the gas actually come from anyway?

— Mostly from bacteria in your gut.

— Hey, I'm clean!

— I'm sure. Look, everybody has bacteria in their intestines.

— Really?

— Indeed. About half the volume of an average bowel movement is bacteria.

— Jesus! How can we get rid of them?

— Usually we don't want to get rid of them, although we could with antibiotics and other drugs. But even though intestinal bacteria sometimes cause problems, others are our best friends. And having the good ones around helps prevent the growth of other bacteria that can cause diar-

rhea. These bacteria do lots of useful things. For instance, we need vitamin K in order for our bodies to produce prothrombin and other factors in the blood which are necessary for clotting. Without clotting we could all bleed to death and without bacteria we'd have no vitamin K because our bodies can't manufacture it and it's not in most people's diet. The bacteria in our digestive system produce it and keep us alive.
— And we keep them alive too.
— Right. From our point of view we're eating to keep ourselves alive. We digest as much as we can in the stomach and small intestine and the broken down nutrients get absorbed through the lining of the small intestine right into our blood stream so that they can be carried away for use or storage. But whatever we can't digest goes on into the large intestine— which is essentially a device for extracting water so it can be recycled in us and reused.
— How ecologically and politically correct!
— Indeed. But something else happens in the large intestine: the bacteria get their meals from our leftovers. As far as the bacteria are concerned, we're there to deliver food to them, but as far as we're concerned, they're there to help us. This arrangement works out just fine for all concerned. It's called mutualism, or, more specifically, symbiosis.
— But what does vitamin K have to do with gas?
— Everything. The bacteria can produce vitamin K because they have enzymes, chemicals that facilitate its manufacture, that we don't have. Likewise, they have enzymes that aren't present in our digestive juices and they can break down chemicals that we can't. They can make a meal out of complex sugars called oligosaccharides. We can't digest them at all, but the intestinal bacteria can break oligosac-

charides down into simple sugars like glucose, which we can digest.
— And then we get the sugar?
— I'm afraid not. The oligosaccharides aren't broken down until the food mass — called a bolus — reaches the large gut, where there's not enough intestinal lining through which to absorb the sugars.
— So, what happens to them? Do they come out with our, uh....
— Stool?
— Stool.
— No. The bacteria keep right on working and break the sugars down further.
— So where's the problem?
— Well, this particular breakdown is called fermentation.
— Like in making wine?
— Like in making champagne.
— With bubbles?
— With bubbles.
— I see.
— So even if you never swallowed any air at all, you still would make some gas, and maybe more than you have to.
— And if that gas got trapped in a bend, then you'd have problems.
— Exactly.
— But my problem isn't pain. I just fart too much.
— Well, there is gas and there is gas.
— You mean there are differences among farts?
— Of course! How do you think I got to be a specialist? There's a great deal to learn about gas in the digestive tract.
— What the hell. We haven't even gotten into Queens yet. I'm game. What's in a fart?

It's a Gas

— Well, let's take it from the top. By sticking tubes in people's stomachs, we've found that gas in that region is pretty much like the air all round us, that is, about 79 percent nitrogen, a gas that isn't absorbed well by the intestines, about 17 percent oxygen, a gas used in many body processes and mostly absorbed from the intestinal tract, and about 4 percent carbon dioxide, formed when the digestive juice from the small intestine meets the stomach acid.

— That's nice, but how does that relate to the gas that comes out the other end?

— Well, if you stick a tube in someone's intestine you'd find...

— How could you do that?

— By shoving it up his....

— No kidding? And I thought cabbies had to take gas.

— Believe me, it's easier with a syringe. Then you can use gas chromatography to analyze intestinal gas and when we do this we find great variation from one individual to another. And the differences are very important.

— For example?

— Well, the collected gas — flatus we call it in the books — is 99 percent made up of five gases: nitrogen, oxygen, carbon dioxide, hydrogen, and methane. Since nitrogen, for example, is not released by the body's own actions or by the actions of bacteria, a fart with a high nitrogen content must have gotten itself started by air swallowing.

— You mean I should collect my farts in a plastic bag and bring them to my doctor?

— I don't think so. Most physicians won't take a sample of bowel gas and if they did it wouldn't matter because most medical labs can't handle it. So the best thing is probably to resort to tests that are less fool-proof but easier to perform.

— For example?

— The easiest test is to look in the toilet after you move your bowels. If you have floating stools, then there's gas trapped in them.

— No shit.

— It's true: floating stools float because of tiny little trapped farts.

— I once picked up a medical student at the morgue who told me that floating turds meant that you had too much fat in your blood.

— I'll bet he did. Passing fat through the system, steatorrhea, is a real problem for people who can't digest fat, but it doesn't show up in floating stools, although most doctors used to think so. Research in this field has only recently been taken seriously enough to get useful results.

— You mean he was wrong?

— Sure. Doctors are human too.

— I know. I had to take this guy to an all nude bar. So what *do* floating turds mean?

— It usually means that your bacteria are producing methane — which is normal in those people who produce it.

— Methane? You mean like natural gas, the kind you use at home.

— Precisely.

— So *that's* where the smell comes from.

— Not so. Methane, as well as oxygen, hydrogen, carbon dioxide and nitrogen, is odorless. Your gas stove smells because the gas company adds smell to the fuel so you won't be able to leave it on by mistake after the flame goes out.

— You mean farts, uh, flatus, really do burn?

— They do, for about one-third of all adults. Now, if you have floating stools you probably produce methane and frankly there's nothing you can do about it. Although this condition isn't inherited, it does run in families who seem to share the same methane-producing bacteria in their colons. Kids raised in families where both parents produce methane are themselves methane producers in 95 percent of the cases while kids raised in families where neither parent is a methane producer only produce methane in about 5 percent of the cases. Of course, all normal flatus after a bean meal contains flammable hydrogen gas.

— How do you know if your floating stools come from methane?

— Easy enough: collect your farts in a plastic bag just the way you said and then, very carefully, try to light them. If they ignite with a blue flame, it's methane.

— Honestly?

— Honestly. But remember to use the plastic bag to separate you from your fart. If you try to light it directly, as many adolescents have tried, you can wind up with some awfully painful burns.

— I know.

— Well, if you do produce a lot of flammable gas and have electrosurgery, say for the removal of a polyp in the colon, you can actually explode. A few people have been injured that way and at least one patient died that way before doctors were aware of the possibility.

— Talk about freak accidents! I remember once on the Long Island Expressway when some yo-yo with MD plates ran right up this Miata's exhaust pipe and....

What's in a Fart?

— Look, that's not the same kind of medical accident. Anyway, nowadays before electrosurgical procedures in the abdominal regions we make sure you skip meals for a while beforehand and then make sure you get a good thorough enema. And aside from electrosurgery, methane is almost never a problem. Since you can't stop producing it anyway...

— What do you mean, "almost?"

— Well, you see, the gases produced in the intestines can pass into the blood stream and the gases in the blood stream can pass into the intestines, as long as they exist in different concentrations. Therefore, since there's no methane normally in the blood stream, some of any methane produced in the gut will pass into the blood. In the same way, the concentrations of gases in the blood and in the air are equalized in the lungs.

— So?

— So if you're producing a lot of methane in your gut some of it is bound to get into your blood; and if you've got a lot of methane in your blood, some of it is bound to get into your lungs. The same with hydrogen. That's why most research in this field measures breath hydrogen. It's easy to collect.

— Does it mean that if my stools float, I shouldn't exhale too close to an open flame?

— No. The concentrations of methane in the breath are usually much too low to burn, but they can allow researchers to check you for methane without putting tubes into uncomfortable places. But, again, that's a complicated test.

— That's a relief! I was beginning to imagine another reason why I shouldn't smoke.

— Well, there is one other rare possibility — but it has happened.

11

— What is it?

— Sometimes a fistula develops, a connecting tube, between the large intestine and the stomach, a sort of extra tube. If you're a methane producer and happen to have a gastric fistula the methane may well back up into your stomach.

— Does that mean that I shouldn't belch near a candle?

— I really wouldn't worry about a gastric fistula. It usually takes an injury or other damage to the stomach and colon to produce one.

— I think I've got the picture on methane. What about the other gases in farts?

— Well, as I said, there's oxygen, but never more than 2 percent of the gas volume. This active element is used by both your own body and by some bacteria in digestion and isn't released by any of them, so the 2 percent we sometimes find is just what's left over from the 21 percent atmospheric oxygen that might have gotten into the gastrointestinal tract through air-swallowing.

— What about the hydrogen and carbon dioxide? Does it matter if you have lots of them?

— Yes, in most people who pass more than normal amounts of flatus, that flatus contains mostly carbon dioxide and hydrogen.

— What's "more than normal?"

— Normal is 400 to 2,000 milliliters a day, between a pint and a half gallon. The amount varies from person to person and in the same person depending upon what he eats.

— You mean like beans?

— That's one thing, sure. Beans are among the foods that contain high percentages of oligosaccharides.

— What are the others?

What's in a Fart?

— Probably just what you'd guess: Brussels sprouts, cabbage. In one study, five hundred people ranked foods in order of decreasing potency as onions, cooked cabbage, raw apples, radishes, beans (which were only fifth!), cucumbers, milk, rich foods, melons, cauliflower, chocolate, coffee, lettuce, peanuts, eggs, oranges, tomatoes, and strawberries. In another study people swore off — or at — broccoli, peas and kohlrabi as well. You can try cutting down on these to decrease gas volume.

— That's just great, but I'll also starve to death.

— Not necessarily, Everyone's intestinal bacteria are individual. You might find that navy beans are your problem but you can get away with melons. Experiment. And while you're experimenting, you can take comfort in one study that demonstrated with great accuracy that while both raisins and apple juice double gas output and bananas increase it by 50 percent and grape juice increases it by 20 percent, both apricot nectar and orange juice are completely safe.

— That's terrific. What about prune juice?

— They tried that too, but it created another condition that made taking the gas measurements rather too difficult.

— I can understand. But stop with all this scientific stuff: the *amount* of gas isn't really the problem. I want tips from my fares. I'm worried about the smell. Which of these gases do I have to cut out?

— Actually, none of them. All five major gases in flatus are odorless. But things get interesting in that little one percent that contains all the other gases of flatus. These fall into six categories and all six smell.

— Now we're getting down to my problem.

— It's not just your problem. Everybody's in the same boat.

13

It's a Gas

— Just so long as they're not all in my cab.

— Don't be so fastidious. This is all a perfectly normal matter of chemistry. The smells come from combinations of small amounts of ammonia, hydrogen sulfide, indole, skatole, volatile amines and short-chain fatty acids.

— That's terrific!

— Okay, let's take them one at a time. Ammonia is often a by-product of the digestion of the amino acids which make up protein, things like meat, fish, eggs and so on. Also from the digestion of glutamine which is found mostly in wheat.

— You mean if my farts smell like window cleaner, I should stop eating those foods?

— Nobody's flatus smells like window cleaner. Ammonia is just one of the sources of odor and may just add pungency to the odor. Besides, there's hydrogen sulfide which comes from foods, especially proteins which contain sulfur and smells like rotten eggs, and there are volatile amines which also mostly come from protein breakdown.

— If I give up meat and eggs, would my smell go down and my tips go up?

— Maybe, but you'd still have skatole and indole to contend with. Skatole is a very special molecule. Its name comes from the Greek word *skatos*, which means *shit*. And that's what it smells like. In fact, skatole is the particular molecule that give feces its characteristic aroma. Indole, which has a similar chemical structure and very nearly the same smell, is usually produced whenever skatole is.

— And when is that?

— Whenever you eat tryptophan.

— What??

— Tryptophan. It's an amino acid, one of the twenty-one building blocks of all the proteins in your body, and in

14

almost all protein-containing foods as well, like eggs and fish and meat.

— Wait a minute. Can't the body make one kind of stuff into other kinds of stuff?

— Definitely. It does that all the time. But there are eight amino acids, and tryptophan is one of them, that the body can't synthesize. They're called essential amino acids and in this case it means that essentially people have to smell.

— I'll just cut out protein.

— That would do it, you're right. Of course, sooner or later you'd die of protein deficiency, but you'd go out smelling like roses.

— If business doesn't pick up, I'll consider it.

— Look, don't try to cut out protein completely from your diet. Everyone really needs it. But if you want to cut down on the smell somewhat, then try cutting down on the protein and building up on the vegetables.

— Do vegetarians smell less?

— They usually do, but remember, plants have proteins too and you have to be careful about foods with lots of oligosaccharides. These don't contribute to smell, but they add lots of carbon dioxide to the flatus and act like a propellant in an aerosol can.

— So let's see. It means that to smell clean, I have to reduce my protein and stay away from oligosaccharides. That doesn't leave much except for water and fats.

— I hate to be so pessimistic but you'll have to watch out for the fats also. Remember those short-chain fatty acids I mentioned? In all of us, some of the fatty acids, or breakdown products of lipids, are not completely absorbed and pass into the colon where the bacteria break them into smaller molecules, the short chain fatty acids, which smell like rancid butter.

— That doesn't leave much except water.

— I'd recommend that you don't try to eliminate all the smell. I think you'll be much better off trying to reduce the volume of your flatus by reducing your oligosaccharide intake. But if you think that your volume of flatus is generally above the normal amount, then there is one common condition you should know about which produces lots of flatus and which is really simple to test. That's lactase deficiency.

— Lactase deficiency?

— The predominant carbohydrate in milk is called lactose. In a normal person this lactose is broken down into two simple sugars, glucose and galactose, by the action of an enzyme called lactase. Most people have lactase in their digestive juices. But if you manufacture little or no lactase, then the lactose from milk or cheese or ice cream passes right down into your large intestine where bacteria go to work digesting it. Not only do they produce lots of carbon dioxide and hydrogen in the process, but they also ferment some of the lactose to short-chain fatty acids. So if you notice that you have more flatus and that it smells worse after you consume milk or dairy products, you may have lactase deficiency.

— Jesus Christ, Doc! That's me exactly! Last week I ate a whole quart of butter pecan and I had to keep the windows open for two days. This is terrific! Now that I know the problem, what's the cure?

— The easiest thing to do is just cut out milk and milk products to see what happens. If that helps with the gas you might want to try acidophilus milk — available in most supermarkets — to see if you can tolerate that. To be even more sure, you could go to a doctor to confirm the lactase deficiency. Although the doctor can't cure it, there's a good test for it called the Lactose Tolerance Test and if you're going to cut out lots of dairy products on a permanent basis, it may be a good idea to make sure that you have lactase deficiency before you do.

— This has got to be a very rare condition.

— Quite the contrary; lactase deficiency in varying degrees is comparatively common and sometimes it's accompanied by abdominal cramps and diarrhea as well.

— Could I have lactase deficiency?

— Anyone *could* have it. Although it is highly unusual before puberty, for adults lactase deficiency is really comparatively common. Probably about one in five adults has it to some degree. Lactase deficiency is clinically present in about 5 percent of the adult white population, and in the non-white population, at least among Americans, the rates have been reported from 60 percent to 90 percent. But the best way to tell if this applies to you is to cut out dairy products and see if you can close your windows more frequently.

— But I love ice cream!

— Well, you could try substituting non-dairy products, like Tofutti, or different brands of frozen yogurt. The lactobacillus in yogurt — and in buttermilk too for that matter — pretty much breaks down the lactose for you so that it never gets to those bacteria in your bowels.

— Come on, Doc! Yogurt instead of cherry vanilla! You've got to have some drug I could take. What about the tablets with whatjamacallit, simethicone?

— Simethicone is an anti-foaming agent. It helps little bubbles get together to make big bubbles. If the problem is in the stomach, it may help you to belch, but it won't cut down your flatus.

— Are there any other medicines?

— Well, some people are helped by taking medicinal charcoal.

— It really works?

— Occasionally. Medicinal charcoal — *never* to be confused with barbecue charcoal — is safe to take and it doesn't require a prescription. Just take a few tablets or teaspoonfuls, depending on the form, with every meal. The charcoal should absorb some of the gas in the gut.

— That sounds just right for me.

— If it works for you it probably is, but charcoal has a tendency to change the stool from brown to black. Most people know that a black stool is often a sign of internal bleeding. It also interferes with absorption of medicines, vitamins, and minerals. So if you take charcoal, don't panic at what comes out the other end.

— But surely there's a wonder drug that will control gas.

— Well, although there's no controlled study to support these claims, some physicians, along with numerous old wives, believe that a vile concoction called asafetida is helpful. And maybe it is. But it isn't manufactured or sold in the U.S.

— Come on, Doctor. You people always have *some*thing you can do.

— There is, at least if the problem is with beans — though we haven't tested it on people with lactase deficiency. There is a drug called Vioform, a bacteriostatic agent. That means that it keeps the bacteria from multiplying and producing gas. And if they don't produce gas, you don't either.

— So give me a prescription for some. *I'll* be the one to test it on lactase deficiency.

What's in a Fart?

— I really don't want to do that.

— Hey, you doctors take too much on yourselves. I ought to be able to make decisions like this for myself. What if I decided to take you to LaGuardia Airport instead?

— Okay, look, Vioform works. And if it should sometime happen that you've just been feasting on bean dip and cheese spread and then discover at the last minute that you have to appear for an emergency audience with the Pope, just give me a call and I'll rush right over with a prescription. Otherwise, I think not.

— Why not, damn it?

— Because gas just isn't a big enough problem. Vioform has been used to cure amebic dysentery — which can be fatal.

— So let it cure gas.

— Oh, it cures gas all right. A number of studies have shown that. But the side effects of the drug are nausea, vomiting, headache, itching and, in a select group with allergic reasons to it, skin rash.

— Well what about antibiotics? They're safe and they kill bacteria. Wouldn't they help?

— Not really. Some studies examining the effects of antibiotics have shown that killing bacteria actually *increases* the volume of gas. You can't kill all the bacteria and apparently the bacteria that are left are usually less efficient digesters, and therefore produce even more gas as waste products. And besides, antibiotics have many other serious side effects and should only be used to treat serious conditions.

— To a lot of people, gas is serious. I wonder what kind of tip *you'll* give me.

— I'll give you two tips: Lactaid and Beano. The first cuts out almost all lactose problems and the second cuts bean gas in half.

19

— That's great! Where do I get this stuff and how do I use it?

— You get it at a pharmacy and if you want to know how to use it, you might read the last chapter of *It's a Gas* by Rabkin and Silverman.

— You've *got* to be kidding.

— Oh, I'm not kidding. Gas is a serious matter. In fact, Hippocrates, the father of medicine, thought that all disease came from gas excreted into various body organs from partially digested food. At least that's how Aristotle's pupil Meno reported the theory. And Antonio Benivieni, the first doctor to seek internal causes of symptoms by autopsy, reported a case in the late 1400s where he concluded that "ex solo vento mors subsequuta," death followed from wind alone. But nowadays in medicine farts are not used much as important signs except after surgery. Right after abdominal surgery, for example, the digestive tract usually becomes temporarily paralyzed; it's a reaction to being directly touched. After the operation the doctors can't administer any fluids or food through the mouth unless they know that the digestive system is functioning again. So they wait for that first fart: it's a crucial sign that post-operative recovery is underway.

— Maybe you could use farts as a sign of other things, like getting the CIA to work out farterprints.

— Farterprints?

— You know, like fingerprints. If a guy eats the same stuff all the time and doesn't take antibiotics, then his gas'll give him away.

— I really don't think so. Too many variables. At least, as far as I know there's no security research into the subject. In

20

fact, much of the interest in fart research doesn't even concern medicine but agriculture.

— Why? Do farmers eat a lot of beans?

— I don't know if they do or don't, but I do know that they raise cattle.

— So?

— Well, in order to take a little calf and grow it into a marketable cow you have to feed it. The food that goes in provides energy with which the cow builds itself up to weight. A lot of that energy is released as methane either through the breath or as farts.

— Cow farts!

— Yes, cow farts. Look, back around 1980 a cow in Holland was being examined by candlelight, farted, and the resulting flame ignited some hay and finally burned down the barn. Cow farts have methane and that's natural gas with a vengeance. About 7 percent of the energy value of cattle food gets blown away.

— I see what you mean. Feed costs money.

— It sure does. And think of the gas! If we could only collect cow belches and farts, which is, I'll admit, a bit difficult, the cattle population of the United States would provide enough gas to supply the household needs of the human population of New York City, Chicago, Los Angeles, Philadelphia and Detroit.

— Just from cows?

— Absolutely. Every damn cow produces gas in the first two of its four stomachs and produces it to the tune of a thousand liters a day, about three hundred gallons. And a quarter of that comes out as farts. In addition, the gas can form as little bubbles causing a disease called bloat. If the animal can't be induced to belch by using foaming agents

21

the farmer has a simple choice between a surgical procedure to let out the gas or a dead cow.

— My god, and I thought I had problems!

— Animal problems with gas are really bad. That's why there's so much research being done on it.

— Can agricultural research help humans too?

— In some ways. Besides the medical techniques for diagnosing and alleviating gas problems, there have been attempts made to create a clean bean that won't cause gas— and it seems to be working.

— Where can I buy some?

— You can't, but the research is really going on right now. And maybe it should because, all kidding aside, gas may be a much bigger problem than anyone ever gives it credit for.

— How is that?

— Well, according to the theory of one doctor, and I'll admit that people haven't all agreed to this yet, holding in farts can be fatal.

— That's damned hard to believe. I hold my gas all the time. I have to. I'm not dead.

— No, you're quite alive. But over the years the building up of gas pressure in the large bowel can have bad consequences. There's the case of one unfortunate boy who pressed a compressed air nozzle to his rectum. Even though he was fully dressed the increased pressure was enough to rupture his colon.

— My God!

— Indeed. Consider this very interesting theory. There is a condition called diverticulosis. It's fairly common and what it means is that there has been "outpouching" in the large intestine, making extra bulges along the walls of the bowels. Now it turns out that city folk get a lot of diverticulosis

22

while country folk, outdoorspeople and so on, rarely do. The theory is that our own inhibitions about breaking wind cause us to hold ourselves in, build up pressure, and thus get diverticulosis.

— Is that so bad?

— Yes, because foodstuff that accumulates in those pouches, just like foodstuff in the appendix, stagnates and you can develop one hell of an infection. When that happens you have diverticulitis, and that can be fatal.

— God damn! Look, Doc, you've convinced me. I *can* cut it down and I will, if not to save my tips then to save my life.

— That's the right idea.

— But speaking of tips, here we are.

— Thank you. It was a very pleasant drive.

— I liked it too.

— Good day.

— Hey, what about my tip!

— What about my bill?

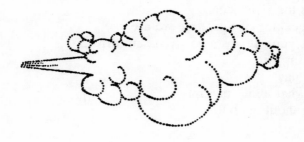

CHAPTER TWO

By Any Other Name
— a linguistic compilation —

The Greeks Had a Word For It.

Zöe Akins, 1930

If there is any form of wind that has more regularly caught humankind's attention than the fart, it is the spoken word. The word *fart* is therefore of double interest. Although this word is now, in the decorous language of the editors of the *Oxford English Dictionary*, "Not in decent use," *fart* was very much an accepted part of Standard English from the thirteenth century to the middle of the eighteenth century, as the epigraphs in this book make clear. But the history of this venerable word is much older than that, and much richer.

By learning how words and languages have developed, and by tracing these developments backwards, linguists have been able to determine that many languages as apparently different as Portuguese and Sanskrit share common roots. Indo-European is the name given to our reconstruction of the prehistoric language which finally gave rise to numerous modern languages including Portuguese, Sanskrit and English among many others. In Indo-European, the word for *fart* is *perd* and this emerged as the Latin *pēdere*, "to fart," and *pēditum*, "a fart." The *p* in these Latin forms becomes an *f* in Germanic and that *f* carried over into English, just as the Latin *pater* became German *Vater* (pronounced fáh-tair) and

25

English *father*. Through a similar process, the *d* in the Latin became a *t*, just as the Latin word *duo* emerged as the English *two*. Hence the Indo-European *perd* became the English *fart*.

Language change, however, is not a simple phenomenon. Sometimes, for example, a word is borrowed into a language at two different times and hence the same word has two different forms as well as two different meanings in the borrowing language. For example, the English *corn*, meaning "a hard protuberance on the foot," is a borrowing from the Latin *cornu*, which we had earlier borrowed but later changed and thus produced the English *horn*, "a hard protuberance on any part of the body" (as in "cuckold's horns" or "horny hands" — two clearly related ideas). Thus words that are apparently quite unrelated may well have been related once upon a time. Similarly, no single law of linguistic change is absolute. For example, not all Latin *d* sounds become English *t*, as we see in English by the light of *day* and in Latin by the light of *dies* (although we find the German *Tag*). Another complication is that sometimes the relations we think we perceive in words aren't really there at all. For example, the Latin *fēci*, meaning "I made, did" is clearly related to the Latin *feces* which we have adopted directly into English as a synonym for the native word *shit*. This may well seem to offer insight into the English slang *doody*, meaning "shit" (as in "Make a doody"), but in fact the English slang comes from "Do your duty" with a softening of the *t* such as we find in many people's pronunciation of such words as "thirty." In other words, with linguistic matters as complicated as they are, it won't do for us to try to discover for ourselves the word relationships that bear on *fart*. But if we're willing to take the results of linguistic research on faith alone, we will catch wind of some surprising things.

26

The Indo-European *perd* led to a Greek *perdomai*, "fart," and took on a related Greek form *perdix* to refer to a type of bird that made an explosive sound when suddenly "flushed." In America a comparatively common related bird is the ruffed grouse. The Greek *perdix* became the Old French *perdriz* and the Modern French *perdrix*. Middle English borrowed the Old French *perdriz* and turned it into *partrich* which comes down to Modern English as *partridge*, the Old World relative to the ruffed grouse. Seeing the etymological connection between *partridge*, and hypothetically, a *fartridge*, we now may have a somewhat better idea of what the bird has been doing in the pear tree all these years.

In an Indo-European variant of *perd*, namely *pezd*, we have the probable source of the Latin *pēdis*, louse, which we have taken into medical English in such forms as *pediculosis*, "infestation by lice." Presumably the louse was associated with a foul smell on unclean people or was itself thought to be foul smelling. At any rate, just as we see *fart* and a bird related in both English and French to a common source, so in Latin we see *pēdere* and an insect related through their common source.

Latin *pēdere* also produced the Latin *pēditum*, "a fart" and this in turn gave rise to the French word for "fart," *pet*. This noun was logically extended to a verb form, *péter*, "to fart," and from that to a whole series of words including *peteur*, "a male farter"; *peteuse*, "a female farter"; and *péterade*, "a series of farts made by a kicking animal." Perhaps the most interesting adaption is *pétard*, meaning "a firecracker" and later "a small bomb used to breach a wall or gate." In its meaning as an engine of war, not as a cracker, it was borrowed into English and is now usually encountered only through Shakespeare's *Hamlet* where we find the expression *Hoist with his own pétard* which has come to mean simply "injured by one's own cleverness." In the original passage, Hamlet gloats over his expectation that his father's murderer will be exposed by his own devices. Those lines take on added significance when we realize the hidden associations of the words:

> Let it work;
> For 'tis the sport to have the engineer
> Hoist with his own petard; and't shall go hard
> But I will delve one yard below their mines
> And blow them to the moon.

> (Act 4, sc 1, 11. 205-210)

Despite its broad and ancient pedigree, *fart*, like so many other words that refer to the bodily functions of sex and elimination, has been repressed in polite English usage. That repression, of course, doesn't mean that the word is no longer part of our language. On the contrary, because the word *fart* is thought of as indecent, its very indecency allows it to be used when a speaker wants to express aggression, just as a fart itself is often taken to be insulting. In addition, because it is somewhat forbidden, it adds a risqué odor to newly coined expressions which can, like aggressive insults, often slip into our language as slang:

28

IMPOLITE IDIOMS

Fart about — this is a mild expression meaning "to dawdle or waste time," a sort of scatological version of "blow an afternoon."

Fart-arsed mechanic — this British expression for "a clumsy person" captures an upper-class disdain for working-class people, as if the upper-classes had "arses" that didn't fart just as much.

Fartarsing about, fartassing around — British and American expressions meaning "driving without a definite idea of one's location," the obvious corollary of "follow the wind."

Fart-catcher — at first meaning "footman" or "valet," this contemptuous reference to someone who *must* follow behind came also to mean, disparagingly, "homosexual," perhaps on the assumption that such an orientation meant that one *wanted* to approach from behind.

Fart in a bottle — this expression uses the off-color associations of fart to refer humorously to someone "flustered" or "agitated." It is supposed to express restless movement, as do the associated expressions, "In and out like a fart in a colander" and "Rushing around like a fart in a colander — doesn't know which hole to come out." (That particular type of entrapment may call to mind an expression proverbial since the 1930s, "a fart's the cry of an imprisoned turd.")

Farting clapper — this synonym for the even more forbidden term "asshole" is one of the rare occasions when the use of the word *fart* is an effort at increased politeness.

Farting Fanny — according to Partridge (not the bird but the editor of the excellent *Dictionary of Slang and Unconversational English*), this name refers to a German heavy gun operating in the Arras sector of France during World War I and also to the shells fired by the gun. Partridge gives this quote: "The War was trundling on quite peaceably as they walked and jogged eastwards towards it, with the occasional clang of Farting-Fanny's arrival in cavernous Arras." Partridge doesn't mention whether "Fanny" has any particular association in this context but surely someone will get to the bottom of it.

Farting shot — a term for an action designed to show contempt for a group as one leaves, probably meant to call to mind "parting shot."

Fart-sucker — a "parasite" or "toady." This phrase is clearly related both to "fart-catcher" and to sundry phrases expressing how far one is willing to go in pleasing another, like "ass kisser" and the somewhat milder "brown nose." Also, the term "fart-sucker" may be related to an interesting bit of French slang. The French police, like the American, often refer to an arrested person as a "suspect." However, its French pronunciation, "soos-pay" is the same as that for the words "suce-pet" meaning "sucks fart" and is accordingly preferred by some police in France in order to legitimately express their contempt for

30

criminals without running the risk of being sued by someone wrongly arrested.

Let a brewer's fart — "to have diarrhea." Obviously derived from the consequences of radically altering the nature of the microscopic life in one's bowels.

As much chance as a fart in a windstorm — "having no chance at all." This linguistically powerful expression serves as a clear compensation for the powerlessness it denotes. Related phrases are "Like a fart in a gale," "Like a fart in a blizzard," "Like a fart in a thunderstorm," "Like a fart in a tornado," "Like a fart in a hurricane," and "Pissing in the wind."

Having all these joking and jibing uses in English, it would be small wonder if encounters with *fart* in other languages didn't sometimes — even if wrongly — strike us as funny.

In Danish, for example, *fart* means "speed". From this association with motion, the Danes derive the word that might well sound to our ears like an award for flatulence: *fartscertifikat*. The word actually means "trade certificate."

In Norwegian, a language quite close to Danish, *fart* also means "motion, speed." From this comes a verb, *farte*, "to wander from place to place." Indeed, the word *fart* is common in Norwegian, in compounds like *fart plan*, which don't at all mean what they imply to us but rather, in this case, "schedule." Don't be offended by the Norwegian who at the outset of a trip, exclaims "Stop-a-fartin," (Stå på fartin) which means "ready to leave" in English.

Similarly, if, when he is seated in your Detroit behemoth, he refers to a "fart smeller" (farts måler), he is probably not making invidious comparisons to the more economical Scandinavian products, but he is merely referring to your speedometer.

The French word *fart* is clearly borrowed from the Scandinavians and denotes the grease used to lubricate the bottom of skis. "Just watch that Frenchman go! He looks like he's racing down that hill on a fart!" Something like American "greased lightning," one supposes.

The Germans also use a word with the same root meaning of motion: *Fahrt*, "journey, trip, tour." American travelers to Germany are probably used to the highway signs, *Einfahrt*, which brings to mind "in-fart" and *Ausfahrt*, which brings to mind "out-fart." These are not doctor's orders, however, but the words for "Entrance" and "Exit." Perhaps more amusing for English speakers, but less well known, are the expressions "wilde Fahrt" and "gute Fahrt!" which mean "going by tramp ship" and "Have a pleasant journey!" respectively.

To the Iberians, *fart* has a totally different meaning. In Spanish a *fart* is "an excess of anything, a glut; especially of food." Perhaps this is related to the nearly identical term for one of the richest of desserts, *farte* meaning "fruit tarte." In Portuguese this last term refers specifically to either a sugar-almond cake or a cream cake. Eating *farts* may not be a very appetizing idea, but eating *fartes* might just be delicious.

And the Italians, of course, sleep in them, since in some dialects *farto* means "mattress."

By Any Other Name

But the Hungarians have the right idea, even though Hungarian is not an Indo-European language. Their word *fartaj* focuses our attention right back where it belongs, on the "buttocks."

Although the association of *fartaj* with "buttocks" is purely fortuitous, an English speaker can often see in other languages the legitimate source of their words for fart.

In Afrikaans, for example, the noun is *maagwind* (clearly, "make wind") and *skeet*, related to our Germanic *shit*. Yet a third term is *poep*, close to the English *poop*. And the verb, *windlet*, is cognate with our "let wind." So perhaps this airy discourse, just like music, is an international language.

In any event, in case you're ever caught somewhere around the world and find yourself with a sudden need to prevent diverticulosis, we present herewith a partially annotated list of nouns, verbs and adjectives arranged in alphabetical order. Alas, this easy-to-use appendix is by no means complete. Would that we knew all the words in all the languages! Your comments, additions and refinements are welcome.

Please turn page.

33

INTERNATIONAL PERDIXICON

Afrikaans   (n)   poep, maagwind, skeet
                           (v)   windlet

Albanian   (a)   mfryet ("That's easy for them to say!")

Arabic   (n)   eegayas (with a big sound)
                                   eezarat (with a small sound)
                                   eefessy (big smell but no sound)

(One should take note here, and also below with such languages as Hawaiian, of the widely believed but controversial "Sapir-Whorf hypothesis." This concept in linguistics, named after its two most forceful early proponents, holds that one's language determines one's way of thinking and vice versa. Famous evidence for this is the wealth of different words in Eskimo for different conditions of snow. The assertion is that an Eskimo speaker really sees more kinds of snow than would an English speaker observing the same scene. If this is true, then to English speakers, basically, a fart is a fart is a fart, but to a speaker of Arabic or Hawaiian this is not the case. They see — detect — subtle differences that insensitive English speakers must have pointed out for them.)

Bantu	(n)	lu-suzi
Bobangi	(n)	mokinyā
	(v)	ta monkinyā
Cantonese	(n)	fong
	(v)	fong p'ayee
Cornish	(n)	bram (pl., bremmyn — but no relation to the Bremen town musicians)
	(v)	brammé, vrammé
Crow	(v)	piaky, pi piahi
	(a)	nadmuty, nabubrelý, nafoukaný
Danish	(n)	fis, skid ("grease his skids with *fart*")
	(v)	fise, slå en skid, slippe en vind (cognate with English "let a wind")
Dutch	(n)	scheet, wind
	(v)	een scheet laten, een wind laten
Esperanto	(n)	furzo
	(v)	furzi (since this language is artificial and based on Indo-European roots, one expects cognates — and finds them)
Finnish	(n)	pieru, ilma vatsassa
	(v)	pierra

French	(n)	pet (pronounced "pay," as in "pay through the nose"), vesse (silent but deadly), pet foireux (nervous and wet), pet de maçon ("mason's fart," i.e., leaves mortar), pet de nonne ("a nun's fart" = a pastry that hisses when it hits the grease), pet de negre (a chocolate pastry), prout (children's term, a "boo-boo"), une pétole (fart with a lump)
		peteur (male farter)
		peteuse (female farter)
		pétarade (series of animal farts)
	(v)	péter, lâcher des vesses
Gaelic	(n)	braim, bram (often associated with raisins)
German	(n)	der Furz
	(v)	furzen
Greek	(v)	perdomai
Hawaiian	(v)	puhi'u (audibly)
		hio, pūhihio, 'ohio (silently = revenge on the Midwest?), pī (sputteringly), 'enakoi (foully)
	(n)	pu'u puhi'u (urge to break wind)
		palalē (sound of breaking wind)
	(a)	makani, palani
Hebrew	(n)	nuhfeechah
	(v)	hahfay-ach

| Hungarian | (n) | koz, fing |
| | (v) | fingik, szellent, buzol |

| Indian (Hindi) | (n) | pud |

| Indian (Kannaras) | (n) | gali |
| | (v) | husu |

| Indian (Malayalam) | (n) | poochi |

| Indian (Tamil) | (v) | kasu |

| Indonesian | (n) | kentut, angin busuk |
| | (v) | berkentut |

| Italian | (n) | peto, scor (reggia) |
| | (v) | fare un peto, scor (reggiare), ruttare |

| Japanese | (n) | he, hohi |
| | (v) | hohi suru |

Kikuyu	(v)	thebea, thuria, eruka eruruka (compare with English *eructation*, meaning "belch")
Lamba	(n)	uwususi
	(v)	uwususi

| Latin | (n) | pēditum |
| | (v) | pēdere |

Malay	(n)	kentut, angin, keleput (sound of breaking wind)
	(v)	ter kentut
Norwegian	(n)	fis, fjert
	(v)	fise, fjerte, slippe en fjert, slippe el fis
	(a)	ful av wind

Phillipines   Tagalog, Cebuano, Samar-Leyte Bisayan: utot
Bikol, Pangasinan: atot
Kapampangan, Ivatan: atut
Ibanag: attut
Ilkukano: uttot
Magindanaw: tut

Polish	(n)	pierdzenic, bzdziny, wiatry (wind)
	(v)	perdziec, bzdziec (cf. Russ), puszcac wiatry (release wind)
	(a)	wywolujacy

| Portuguese | (n) | peido, gas intestinal |
| | (v) | expelir gases intestinais, peidar |

Romanian	(n)	gaze, suflu
	(v)	suflare
	(a)	a avea vênturi

Russian	(n)	perdyozh (act of breaking wind)
		perdun (the outcome, also the perpetrator)
		perdil'nik (the place from whence it comes)
		Perun (the ancient god of wind)

		bzdun, bzdyukha (a silent fart, also a stupid jerk)
	(v)	perdet' (to do it with or without sound) bzdet' (to do it silently); the use of prefixes and suffixes is permitted: pereperdet' (to fart repeatedly, to refart), nabzdet'sya (to fart silently to complete satisfaction)
Slovene	(n)	pezdec, ventrovi
	(v)	pezdeti, ventrovi imeti
Spanish	(n)	pedo, flato (Greek philosophers?)
	(v)	pedorrear, peer, ventosear, tirar un pedo (let one fly)
Swedish	(n)	fjärt
	(v)	släppa sig
Tarahumara	(n)	uii-re
	(v)	uii
Welsh	(n)	gwynt, yn y bol
	(a)	gwyntog, bolwyntog
Yiddish	(n)	nefikhe
Zulu	(v)	suz, shipha

*****

39

It's a Gas

Having winded our way from Afrikaans to Zulu, we've passed full circle linguistically and arrived back at our starting point geographically. The words and euphemisms for fart abound, bursting out here and there and calling attention to themselves in many languages. But, as Shakespeare said:

What's in a name? That which we call a rose
By any other name would smell as sweet.

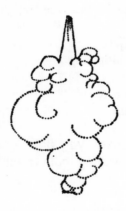

CHAPTER THREE

Wherever the Four Winds Blow
— *an anthropological tour* —

> *What winde can there blowe,*
> *that doth not some man please?*
> *A fart in the blowyng*
> *doth the blower ease.*

John Heywood, 1556

To most members of our well-perfumed culture, flatulence causes but one reaction: we look down our nose at it.

To prevent such disfavored outbursts, Western restaurants often thoughtfully give out peppermints. Peppermints, it turns out, are considered a "carminative." A carminative is a drug which prevents the formation of undue gas in the stomach or bowel, and just as every culture has its own favorite aphrodisiacs, so every culture has its own favorite carminatives. Unfortunately, the carminatives are no more effective than the aphrodisiacs. (Though there is one culture where a carminative, if it worked, would be an *anti*-aphrodisiac — but that's for later.) In fact, the reason that you'll find peppermints next to the cash register in so many restaurants is not so you can save money on the dessert but so that you can "aid digestion." Principally, that means cutting down instead of cutting loose. As you travel around the world, whenever you hear a fart, watch what people grab. Somewhere or other people will use cloves, nutmeg, cinnamon, lemon, pepper, ginger, cardamom, oil of lavender, aniseed,

41

coriander, dill or gentian as carminatives. And, of course, peppermints. According to this way of thinking, if you've been drinking herb tea or stoking up on kosher pickles, you ought to be as windless as the eye of a hurricane.

Unfortunately, none of this seems to work. Since stomach eruptions are primarily caused by air swallowing, digestion isn't even a relevant problem — chewing and swallowing are the culprits. As for the real thing down below, none of these remedies has any value at all. No "aid" to the digestion will help you to improve the impression you've been making on the person who sits at the desk just downwind. But all these scientific facts don't mean that people the world over haven't tried to tame the wild fart. Every culture has its own ideas. A little honest investigation will quickly prove that "beauty is in the nose of the beholder." As Hamlet said, "There is nothing either good or bad but thinking makes it so." So in this chapter we will examine the thinking of people round the world and see what they might do instead of beholding the nose.

The Burmese, for example, have an interesting set of beliefs about farting. In *Alice in Wonderland* the caterpillar explained about eating his mushroom: one side would make Alice grow, the other would make her shrink. Finally she decided to carry pieces from each side of the mushroom in pockets on either side of her apron. Then, whenever she wanted to change heights, she would nibble her uppers and downers alternately until she got to be just the size she wanted. In Burma cucumber is thought to be *lay-hto-ti*, meaning that it brings on flatulence. (No wonder there's not much market for kosher pickles in Burma!) On the other hand, citron is *lay-naing-ti*, meaning it "conquers wind." So when a guest happens to drop in they serve up a *to-sa-ya* plate, with cucumber on one side and citron on the other. Then, like Alice, the lucky devil can nibble here and nibble there until just the right friendly atmosphere is established.

The Devil is not to be taken lightly in matters of flatulence. Martin Luther believed, on the basis of personal experience, that farts could scare away Satan himself, so in the case of infernal temptation, you might want a little *lay-hto-ti*.

"Merde du Diable" in French and "devil's dung" in English are alternate terms for the word "asafetida," referring both to a certain plant of the genus *Ferula* and to the brown, sticky, vile-smelling gum made from this and related plants. In medieval Europe, if someone were bewitched, the prescribed cure for the spell was to wash the person's arms and legs in his own urine. If the solution proved too weak, it would be strengthened by the addition of asafetida. Perhaps this is what was meant by the phrase "stink to high heaven!"

The people of central Thailand forbid milk-giving women from eating jackfruit because it causes excessive gas, and in the eyes of those beholders excessive gas is no laughing matter. They believe that flatulence can result in blindness or even death and that smells, which they consider air-borne foods, are to be avoided since they worsen wind excess. The Thais use asafetida as a carminative. When a baby has excessive gas, since he can't help himself, the Thais tie some asafetida to the helpless little wrist in the hope that the devil's dung will set the devil to rout. However, considering the aroma that lends asafetida its damnable nickname, one cannot help wondering if the poor little devil is being subjected to a cure that is considerably worse than the disease. If only his parents could simply take a philosophic attitude toward his flatulence and comfort themselves with the thought that "This too will pass."

Unfortunately, they could not ignore such a condition. When the fart is heard round the world, most noses wrinkle and most people are offended. Although the reaction to intestinal gas may be either mild or extreme, generally speaking, as in America, efforts are made to conquer it. We find particularly mild measures among the Fellahin of the northern Egyptian deserts. These people feel that farting is offensive and try not to do it, but ignore it in children under the age of about ten. Once children, especially boys, reach this age, their playmates gently train them not to fart. If a fart is cut during group play, they will question each other to discover the culprit and if the offender denies his transgression, they will smell each other until they discover the guilty one. Obviously among children farting is only mildly disapproved and is regarded with some humor. But once the culprit is discovered, for this lie as much as for this fart, he is ridiculed. Because the agemates have such keen eyes — and noses — Fellahin parents can leave this aspect of child-rearing to the *peer* group.

Among the Kaska Nahane, Indians of British Columbia, people follow a ritual of competitive consumption called a "potlatch." Individuals contest with each other for social prestige by seeing who can burn up the greatest quantity of valuable blankets and articles of copper and who can host the most sumptuous feasts. Although farting is repressed in this culture, and children are taught not to do it, especially in the company of adults, nonetheless excessive overeating just naturally leads to excessive build-ups of gas and the Kaska Nahane quite sensibly choose to ignore this aspect of child-rearing during a potlatch. Perhaps it is hard to compete with the smell of burning copper.

An anthropologist who studied the Selkinam people of Tierra del Fuego reports that he once saw a dog who had the misfortune to expel gas in a hut full of people. The animal was immediately driven out by a barrage of stones and sticks. People may or may not be treated somewhat more gently. When someone in a group of Selkinam breaks wind, the whole group breaks up, running around and chasing the offender away. Unless, of course, the offender happens to be a respected elder, in which case most people ignore the offense while others smile in the same way one would at hearing an improper joke. A fart is not a fart is not a fart, it seems, because who does the farting, when, and how makes all the difference in the world.

Among the Toradja of central Celebes, a remote people of Indonesia, farting is considered all right, except that all of the products of the human body are supposed to have magical powers. Thus the circumstances surrounding the fart are all important. Usually it can be simply ignored, but the Toradja believe that farting will bring bad luck if it occurs during certain key activities: gathering clay for pot-making, panning for gold, embarking on a hunt or journey, or leading a bridegroom to the house of this bride. There is no social punishment meted out to the offenders: the bad luck of ruining your own marriage is considered punishment enough.

The Tartar Khans seem to have understood this type of bad luck. Marco Polo reported that when a woman was brought in for consideration as a potential wife, the Khan would first have her sent to live with the wives of his under-lords. If they reported that she neither snored nor farted in her sleep, then she might have a chance of getting into the big time.

45

It's a Gas

The Waleaians of the Caroline Islands make an interesting distinction between locales for farting. To the Waleaians all bodily functions, including defecation, urination, and crepitation, are considered shameful if someone is seen performing them *on dry land*. However, it is perfectly acceptable to do these things *underwater*. For whatever prehistoric reasons of safety against attacks by shark or hostile humans, these people have developed the custom of whole communities performing together their daily ablutions in public in their lagoon where they feel free to void themselves of solids, liquids and gas. But if they were caught releasing so much as a small fart on land, the community would laugh at them thoroughly until they showed great shame.

Farting is no laughing matter in nearby New Guinea. The Kapuaku disapprove of anything coming out of the human body. Some emanations — a cough or belch, for example — are considered to be mildly offensive and result, whether committed by child or adult, in a simple admonition to behave properly. But for willfully indecent acts, and to the Kapuaku these acts include spitting on the floor (instead of into the fireplace), blowing the nose, and farting, adults may be punished by expulsion from the group while children may be beaten with sticks.

Among the Thonga of South Africa, such ritual beating has come to figure in peer-group initiations. Among goatheards, for example, when one of them is detected to have let a fart, they yell *Fakisa* at him — what has happened? Everything is fine if he will just respond simply with the words *Cita munyakanya goben* — I have let my wind out through the rectum. But if he does not know the formulaic admission, he is beaten and made to take over the herding until the end of that day. Things are arranged so that a boy is not very likely

46

to learn the mystic formula until his fellows want him to. First of all, if the formula is revealed to an uninitiated boy the one who reveals it is given the same punishment of beating and being forced to take over the herding. And second, although these people are a Bantu tribe, *Cita munyakanya goben* is a sentence in Zulu. Perhaps this is their way of expressing an opinion of their neighbors.

Among many Arabs, farting is considered to be the single gravest indecency. Some closely knit tribes will make an individual a perpetual butt if he commits such an offense as an adult. Until modern times, among the Belludjages near the Iranian frontier, the result of expelling gas was expulsion from the tribe. Even worse, among the pre-modern Bedawi — who by the way were required by custom to belch in order to express satisfaction at a meal — farting was so despised that should a warrior at an oasis break wind despite himself, and should a bystander happen to laugh, the bystander would be cut down on the spot. This same custom was observed through the nineteenth century among the warrior Highlanders of Afghanistan. Thus, we see that in ancient times both these groups were dominated by the same aggressive pre-Ishmaelite Arab marauders. Who knows what marvelous knowledge we might discover if only we were willing to follow the right scent?

Many pre-European black Africans considered farting to be indecent in the extreme and would go to extraordinary lengths to contain themselves and thus avoid giving insult. Many seventeenth century Dutch trading ship captains remark in their logbooks that the Africans were aghast at the continual and unembarrassed farting of the white sailors, who apparently felt no such inhibition. Even among blacks who accepted farting as natural among themselves, as did some of the groups in Angola, they would never take such license in front of strangers the way the Dutch did. And some groups, of course, were stricter yet. The Ashanti of the Gold Coast (now Ghana) considered public farting a pure disgrace. If a group of Ashanti happened to be eating together and one broke wind the others would degrade him by putting the bowl of food on this head for the remainder of the meal. If the group happened to be good friends, however, all would cover their mouths with their hands to hide their laughter until they could get out of view (outside the hut or behind a bush) because — it has been asserted — they feared that if their friend saw their laughter he would be so mortified that he would go off and hang himself!

The Ashanti are not unique in their mortal hatred of farting. The Trobriand Islanders of Melanesia make it a point of honor never to expel gas in the presence of other people, even if, by virtue of being in a group, they might do so undetected. To a Trobriand Islander all important daily events seem not the result of hard work or luck but of spells cast by someone or spells cast upon one by others. The sense of smell is very important in laying spells on people since magic of the greatest potency is thought to enter through the nose. Thus the casual letting of a fart at the wrong time might ruin a good day's conjuration. Malinowski, the famous anthropologist who first studied these people, comments that because of this inhibition a native crowd is "considerably more pleasant in this respect than a gathering of European peasants." The Trobrianders tell a folk story of a louse, a worthless parasite, who rode a butterfly. Because the louse could not properly control himself, he farted and the recoil of this emission was so strong that the louse was blown off the butterfly's back and into the sea — where he deservedly drowned. Thus are little Trobrianders taught about the kind of people who fart and what becomes of them.

No one, we might imagine, would choose the fate of the louse, and yet there are records of closely allied cases. Among the Tikopia of nearby Polynesia children may freely urinate in public. Within the family circle, men may arise at any time and urinate without restraint. Similarly, a man among his own children, or with a group of young bachelors, may fart as much as he likes. But as the situation changes, the response changes. If a child farts in a mixed group of children and adults, an adult may reprove him while the other children will laugh at him. These actions, in such an informal setting, are mild and no effort is made to camouflage the underlying air of amusement and embarrassment. But in an extremely formal situation, the result of a fart may be extreme indeed. This was so in the case of a young man named Pu Sao. In a gathering of chiefs, Pu Sao quite audibly broke wind. He was overcome with shame and immediately left. Days later he was found at the top of a coconut palm. At the place from which the leaves grow there is usually a spear-like projection, called a spathe, sticking straight up. He had committed suicide by impaling himself through the rectum on such a spathe and bleeding to death.

In the Truk Islands, also in the South Pacific, the *fadanap* is a most solemn occasion in which the tribes gather and their communal food is redistributed to all by the chief of chiefs. Each person immediately consumes whatever he can and the remainder is ceremonially carried back home. As in the case of the potlatch, with so much eating, something has to be brewing. At one such *fadanap* "a young chap let out a noise that filled him with such shame that he went into the forest, reviled his rectum, and ripped it open with a sharp shell, so that he bled to death." These suicides by self-attack against the offending part are clearly symbolic of the degree to which some people, when they hear a fart, feel not annoyance but shame or terror.

The Canelos Indians of Ecuador are particularly scared by farts because they believe that the soul escapes the body along with the smell. They have developed a ritual to counter this escape. When in a group someone breaks wind, one of the rest, the quickest, will clap him on the back three times and say *uianza, uianza*! The meaning of this word is unknown but it does signify a feast by that name which the person who farted is obliged to prepare. After being clapped on the back the farter and the *uianza* shouter join hands and their hands are then separated by a third party, as if they were making a bet. In this way the farter makes his pledge to follow through with the feast. Alternatively, he can discharge his obligation by rewarding the clapper's kindness with three big clay vessels of manioc-beer. Although it seems to us that all the advantage lies with the one quick enough to shout *uianza*, we can understand that the one who farted in the group might truly consider it a kindness if the result of this shouting and feasting is the return of his soul to his body. What we cannot understand — because it has not been reported — is what the Canelos do when they fart alone.

Many groups, like the Canelos, repress farts so strongly that — perhaps to escape the fate of Pu Sao — they have developed rituals that invariably accompany these backward belches. The Thonga, for example, the South African Bantu tribe, hold that a man's relation to his wife's brother's wife is of special importance and this person is known as his Great Mukonwānā. The Great Mukonwānā always looks on a man's farting as a grave offense and should a man commit it in her presence he is obliged to appease her by the payment of a fine, such as a hoe. If the man has nothing on hand with which to make the payment, he breaks a twig from a tree and presents that as a sign that he will pay. Since trees don't grow on water, for fear of being caught short without a fart payment, the Thonga men, even if they must cross a river with their Great Mukonwānā, will not go with them in the same boat. The ritual nature of these actions is clear. Whereas a Westerner caught in such a situation might just carry along an extra twig, the Thonga realize that if the ritual is not performed properly it is worthless. To prepare a twig in advance might well imply that the man planned on farting at his Great Mukonwānā, and premeditated farting is even worse than the accidental kind.

Among the Chagga of Africa we find a ritual that is even more surprising, but perhaps should not seem so in this largely male chauvinist world of ours. To fart among the Chagga is to become ridiculous. It follows, then, by the crazy logic of the sexes, that if a man farts at the dinner table, his wife must pretend that it was she who let fly. In fact, she must allow herself to be scolded about it by the husband. If she doesn't do this, and thus the children have occasion to taunt their father, the wife is required to pay a penalty of three barrels of beer. Since women in such a situation might well resent their roles they sometimes gossip about the indignities they are forced to suffer. A common saying is "Mi aamko ndzoka: moruru adeka kakumba vela katatska" which means "The snake of life rose up in my husband, and it sounded, created waves, and formed drops." This phrase, although common, is obviously disrespectful and should the husband find that his wife has been airing her grievances she is required to pay an even larger penalty of three goats, one to the village elders, one to the husband's male peer group and one to the husband's parents. (Perhaps because this last group includes women, the wife can substitute the lesser fee of a barrel of beer.) Despite the burdensome consequences to the woman, reference to a husband's flatulence occurs regularly. Around the world, whenever an individual who feels himself to be dominated can find no other valve for the release of social pressures upon him, he can at least resort to the mention of forbidden subjects. This is true for children in societies with rigorous child-rearing practices, for working people in societies dominated by wealth, and for women in societies dominated by men.

In our culture, it is still considered indecent in some circles to make any reference whatsoever to the functions of elimination or sex. Because of the anatomical proximity of urethral opening and vagina, and because of the urinary and sexual functions of the penis, most cultures associate elimination and sex. In our culture, because our religious institutions concern themselves with regulation of sexual activity, references to these associated functions are not only obscene but profane. The four-letter words in English are therefore doubly powerful in puncturing propriety. In one statistical study, Vladimir Piskacek observed that swearing is about fifty times more common in the lower classes than in the upper classes. The upper crust, of course, consider this a mark of the worthlessness of their supposed inferiors and, as part of their effort to set themselves apart, cultivate propriety. The people on the short end of the cultural stick, even if unable to achieve economic and political success, can at least reject the restrictive mores of the in groups. Failing that, they can at least verbally re-create the forbidden actions as a last defense against domination.

Freud suggested that many children first rebel against the authority of their parents during the process of toilet training. In all people at some times, and for many people at all times, the anus is an erogenous zone. Freud asserts that some children want to hold back their gas and stool so that they can release it in the biggest and best — and often most private — manner that they can devise, savoring each pleasant sensation. The parent on the other hand wants cooperation and *wants it now*. It is only a few years after this battle of the bottoms that children begin to express their rebellion against their parents by specifically using the forbidden words that refer to the forbidden acts. Although most of us outgrow the need to expel this verbal gas, most of us retain some vestiges of rebellion. They very clearest case of this is the so-called "Bronx cheer," what one psychologist has called "an oral fart," perhaps the most obvious and unspellable negative comment in our language or any other. Dante recognized the connection between the Bronx cheer and the fart in "The Inferno," Canto XXI, lines 137-139 (1321). When the minor devils razz the Devil himself, he answers with the real thing:

> Each with his tongue between his teeth a-stretch
> Made signal to his captain; he, reversed,
> Made suddenly a trumpet of his breech.

When the umpire makes a stupid call — and refuses to see that he is exercising his authority unjustly — then come the Bronx cheers. Precisely because farting is a repressed function the ritual noise has useful psychological effects for the fans who must sit in the bleachers and watch their team lose.

Sometimes the loss is not the temporary outcome of a game but the permanent fact of class differentiation. Americans are uncomfortable with class distinctions. The better off among us, then, have three choices: first, they could devise a plan that would allow the worse off to raise themselves to a better position — this has seemed good to all concerned, but also it has seemed impossible; second, they could redistribute their money and goods so that they were not better off — this has often seemed desirable to the potential recipients, but somehow the rich have never gone along with it in great numbers; and third, the upper classes, while maintaining their position, could make it appear that their position was the same as everyone else's — a solution that may not work forever but which everyone seems to be having a lot of fun trying. The reason is simple: to appear unprivileged in America, all one needs to do is talk dirty, an act that carries out as an adult our repressed childhood rebellion. Lip service to the ideal of equality has become a Bronx cheer. When we say "Everyone's shit stinks just the same," or when the British upper-classes call each other "old fart," the language itself ritually creates a social camaraderie by standing on its head the ritual of breaking bread together. Instead, we break wind together. Psychologist Renatus Hartogs tells of a boss at an advertising firm who always advises newcomers that "you can't be creative all the time. Just work in shits and farts." The man asserts that by playing around with the phrase "fits and starts" and making it into a vulgarism the employees visibly relax and the employee-employer class barrier begins to crumble. Because the particular vulgarity concerns elimination — so often unconsciously associated with sexuality/creation — the joke, though Hartogs does not mention it, is doubly effective in reducing the fear of having to "be creative." The link between the sexual and the eliminative is painfully close in this case. The new men on the job are "scared shitless" but are relaxed when their own private fears are made public by hearing the boss come out with "shits and farts." In such ways, the fact of repression creates the possibility for rituals that may actually benefit society.

The Amhara of the Ethiopian Highlands seem to have understood this. Although they mildly repress discussion of the bodily functions, acceptable outlets exist for the functions themselves. Even in polite society, farting is nearly inevitable among these poor people who subsist largely on roast peas or barley. When someone breaks wind, he will frequently utter this proverb: "The Abyssinian [Amhara] is clever; bowing low [before a great man], he silently farts." The proverb, a verbal ritual, helps the exploited segment of society accept the conditions they must suffer. Thus the initially repressed act becomes almost a preferred act by which the dominated can impose himself on the dominator. In a similar turnabout young girls among the Timbira Indians of the Amazon rain forest in central Brazil will not only acknowledge the pleasant sensations attached to the forbidden act of farting but will go off into the forest together to hold farting contests, even beating their buttocks with their fists in an effort to increase their air power. But, of course, they will not do this with adults present and they no longer indulge (at least in groups) as adults. The Siriono of Peru, on the other hand, indulge in farting whenever possible in groups of two. The intense emotions and activities of intercourse often accelerate flatulence and the Siriono find that farting during coitus is a definite pleasure. They like to couple in hammocks expressly so that the necessary contortions will more readily make their air apparent. Climactic farting is looked upon as a sign of sexual prowess. This glorification of the fart would seem to contrast irrevocably with the Arab detestation of farting. Yet even among the Arabs the fart can be reinterpreted. Niebuhr records a case of a sheik among a tribe called the Montesids who arranged a challenge match for farting among his servants and crowned the winner. By the mock election of the victor to the rank of sheik, one is reminded of the boss of the advertising agency trying to improve productivity by removing the fears attendant on class distinctions.

*****

Since we see that some societies manage to turn farting and the discussion of farting to good social purposes, it should not be too surprising to find cases in which repression is not merely mild but absent. A turn of the century text asserts that among Brahmins there was once an eating ritual that required at the first mouthful saying "Glory to the wind which dwells in the chest"; at the second mouthful, "Glory to the wind which dwells in the face"; at the third mouthful, "Glory to the wind which dwells in the throat"; at the fourth mouthful, "Glory to the wind which dwells in the whole body"; and finally, at the fifth mouthful, "Glory to those noisy ebullitions which escape above and below." More solemnly, medieval Catholics used Saint Erasmus as the intercessor in cases of disorders of "the belly, with the entrayles," making him therefore the patron saint of farts. And Robin Goodfellow, the medieval household sprite who sometimes helped but more often bedeviled the domestic life of the times, was represented as singing this song:

When lads and lasses merry be,
With possets and with juncates fine [curdled milk
  delicacies],
Unseen of all the company,
I eat their cakes and sip their wine;
And to make sport,
I fart and snort,
And out the candles I do blow.

Robin Goodfellow was a medieval invention, originally the name given the supernatural domestic spirit who aided overworked housewives. Apaches in America also had attendant spirits. One of the key rites of passage of the Apache was a lengthy period of isolation. A brave-to-be would go sit out alone on a mountainside where eventually, by sleeplessness, hunger and exposure to the elements, he would finally have a vision. In this vision he would learn which manner of beast would be his familiar, whether a buffalo or a bird or a certain kind of snake. Thereafter in life he could expect supernatural help from members of that species in times of great need. Sometimes a man's familiar would not be alive in the usual sense but might be rain or lightning or the wind. M.E. Opler, who studied the Apache, records one case of a man who claimed that the wind which was his familiar was about as familiar a wind as you can imagine: he claimed to receive supernatural knowledge from his own farts. Numerous informants corroborated this brave's use of his special powers to predict the outcomes of games of chance.

The oldest example of the religious use of farts may be among the ancient Pelusians of northern Egypt who worshipped a fart-god called Bel-Phegor which was idolized as a swollen paunch. The adherents to this sect would offer up excrement and flatulence in gratitude for the good health of which these sacrifices were presumably a sign. (Since the worship of Bel-Phegor was abominated by the ancient Hebrews, the existence of this cult may help explain the meaning of this odd line from the Book of Isaiah: "Wherefore my bowels shall sound like a harp of Moab, and mine inward parts for Kir-haresh" [xvi. 11].) The Eskimos, too, accepted the power of farts. Their god Torngarsuk, a being described alternately as like a great bear, like a great man with only one arm, or as formless, was said to inhabit huts in which witchcraft was being performed. If a fart were cut at times of spell-casting, Torngarsuk would be killed. The Serbs, though Christians, also believed in the destructive power of eructations and viewed excessive gas as a case of possession by a fart-demon. They dealt with the demon, whom they called Matrun, as they did with all possessive demons, by formulaic exorcism. The spell to overcome gas is this: "In the name of the Father, and of the Son and of the Holy Spirit, Amen. I conjure you Matrun! Why do you torment the body of this servant of God? And bellow like a bull, leap like a stag, bark like a dog? I conjure you Matrun to go back to your own place and not to molest the body of God's servant _____." Fill in the blank according to need.

Although the English editions of Martin Luther's "Table Talk" seem to have been expurgated, in the Latin edition he tells of a woman who "Sathanum crepitu ventris fugavit": "sent off the devil by her crackling wind." Perhaps this belief in the efficacy of farts may account either for the practice or the timing of what have been called "obscene tenures." In feudal England and Ireland there were numerous packets of land which required of their holders not only military service to the lord from whom the land was held but "Die Nativitatis Domini coram eo saltare, buccas cum sonitu inflare, et ventrum crepitum edere," "on the Day of the Birth of God, before the lord, publicly to jump, to blow out the cheeks with sound, and to give out the creakings of the belly." One vassal who discharged his duties with particular skill went down in history for his "leap, puff, and fart" as "Baldwin le Peteur," Baldwin the Farter.

A related rental agreement required that the Lord of the Manor of Essington, in order to continue to hold his tenure from the Lord of the Manor of Hilton, had to bring a goose to the hall of Hilton Manor each New Year's Day and drive it around the main hearth at least three times "while Jack of Hilton is blowing the fire." Jack of Hilton turns out to be a brass statue about twelve inches high of a man kneeling on his left knee and holding his erect penis in his right hand. There is a little hole in the mouth of the statue through which water can be poured and when the statue is backed up to the hearth, the heat causes boiling which creates a loud noise and sustained jets from the brass anus. This is indeed a long way from repression.

Perhaps the first would-be law concerning farting is mentioned in the biography of the Roman Emperor Claudius. This kind tyrant had heard of a person who had farted at a public feast and was so overcome by shame that his modesty caused him to gag, nearly killing him. Claudius intended therefore to publish an edict allowing all people to vent their flatulence at table with no penalty. Unfortunately, before this typically sensible judgment of the Emperor's could be promulgated, he ate a dish of poisoned mushrooms thoughtfully served up by his third wife. Perhaps she couldn't stand the idea of what those state dinners might be coming to.

It's a Gas

A somewhat later fart law of interest is that concerning
the French village of Montluc which required that a prostitute
entering the city for the fist time must pay a toll at the bridge
of four denarios or else of one fart. This odd demand may be
related to the widespread medieval belief that the Devil had
a hand in the building of bridges. In order to expiate his
interest and make the bridges safe, human sacrifice was
sometimes used in the early centuries of this era, sometimes
walling infants up in the pediments, sometimes mixing the
mortar of the cornerstone with human blood. We have
already noted the later belief that farts send off the Devil.
Perhaps the toll exacted from prostitutes was considered a
useful, if unseemly, ritual. In any event, knowing of this law
helps make sense of an odd passage in Victor Hugo's *Notre
Dame de Paris* (1832) which we know in English as *The
Hunchback of Notre Dame*. The novel is set in the fifteenth
century. In the very first chapter we encounter a crowd scene:

— Abbé Claude Choart! docteur Claude Choart! Est-ce
que vous cherchez Marie la Giffarde?
— Elle est rue de Glatigny.
— Elle fait le lit du roi des ribands.
— Elle paie ses quartre deniers; *quatuor denarios*.
— *Aut unum bombum.*
— Voulez-vous qu'elle vous paie au nez?

Which translates:

— Abbot Claude Choart! doctor Claude Choart! Are
you searching for Marie la Giffarde?
— She is on Glatigny Street.
— She keeps house for the chief of the camp followers.

— She is paying her four denarios; four denarios.
— Or one explosion.
— Do you want her to pay you through the nose?

The pun comes through in English or French, but the basis for it is only clear when we know the law.

Law, of course, is largely codified custom and belief. Yet despite our obvious modern repression of the subject of farts and despite our far-ranging concern for public sanitation and the rights of others, there seems to be precious little about farts in the law. There is an important civil suit involving Joseph Pujol, but that matter will be reserved for fuller discussion in Chapter Four. There really seem to be no criminal laws, in America at least, concerning farting. The closest one comes to such a law is an anti-smell ordinance like the following: "Persons with offensive odors are not allowed upon streetcars. It shall be unlawful for anyone who has on or about his person any disgusting or offensive smell or odor to board any streetcar in the city of Atlanta for the purpose of becoming a passenger thereon, or for any purpose whatever... when requested to quit said car by the conductor." Now this would make it possible to eject someone who farted while on the streetcar — if the conductor could believe that a fart was necessarily disgusting even though it improves sex and drives off the devil — but as for keeping a farter off to begin with, well, gas will take care of its own: the evidence of past farts is usually gone with the wind.

This failure on the part of our legislators could hardly reflect a failure of imagination. Clearly they must have had something in mind when they made it illegal to sell cabbage on the Sabbath in Ocean City, New Jersey, to eat peanuts in court in Massachusetts, and to divorce a woman in Tennessee without leaving her, among other things, ten pounds of dried beans. These hard working public servants do come awfully close to our subject, having made it illegal to sneeze on the streets of Asheville, North Carolina or on a train in West Virginia, to spit against the wind in Sault Ste. Marie, Michigan or from subway platforms in New York City, to whistle on Sundays in Maine or under water in Vermont, and to snore at night in Coral Gables, Florida. Yet they don't actually come right out and say that farting is illegal. Is it just possible that America is learning to think of this natural function as merely natural, like hiccoughing? After all, the Onge of the Andaman Islands have huge pork orgies that result in extraordinary flatulence, but they are too smart to let the smells interfere either with the eating or the laughter; Brahmins, even when they don't praise the winds of their bodies, may often fart after a meal as heartily as a European will utter a satisfied sigh; and when the Trumai Indians of central Brazil belch or fart they don't think anything of it — unless it smells unusually bad, in which case someone might spit in understandable disgust. Could it be that we are as enlightened as these people we look down our sensitive noses on? Of course not. The reasons we have no laws about farting is that we don't need the customs codified: the customs are working fine all by themselves. Farting is forbidden to young and old alike, in peer groups and in mixed groups, before eating and during sex and after death. And if a fart should, terribly, be heard in our part of the world, we have our ritual all prepared: we may roll the eyes upward as if abstractly examining the ceiling until the smell passes or else we can say firmly and with the weight of social power behind us, "Who cut the cheese?"

CHAPTER FOUR

Good Ole Farts
— a biographical sideshow —

A voice within us speaks the startling word.

Richard Henry Dana, 1833

To mask the sound of an occasional indiscreet release of gas, Victorian women would rustle their bustles. Joseph Stalin, who needed to fear very little, kept a water carafe and several glasses on his desk in part so that his intentionally clumsy clinking of them would camouflage his less memorable utterances from below. But not everyone has shown this modesty. Sometimes even against our wills we must do what we must do, and it is the people who do these things heroically who sometimes make history.

A simple case is that of an unnamed European tailor reported by Drs. Bach and Goldberg. This man, though much sought after by customers, was on the verge of abandoning his profession because of a crucial lack of control. It seemed that nearly every time he bent over to measure the inseam of a client he would fart. This naturally embarrassed the tailor and represented something of a business liability as well. Psychiatrists came to the conclusion that this tailor in fact had a rather overdeveloped cleanliness complex and deeply resented having to touch his patrons' dirty shoes. According to the psychiatric theory, the tailor's uncontrollable farting was actually an unconscious but aggressive reaction against his situation. The most inexpensive expedient was the employment by the tailor of a full-time shoeshine man who cleaned the customer's shoes before each fitting. According to the reporting physicians, the shoeshine man effected an immediate cure.

Aggressive farting may have its conscious uses as well, naturally enough. The position of "court fool" is a strangely complex one. These kept jesters most often were far from stupid, but rather *chose* to appear stupid in order to perform acts and utter notions that, on reflection, showed real appreciation of the subtleties of human affairs. Part of the poignancy of this occupation is that both fool and courtiers knew of the sham but both had to act as if the sham were the truth. The fool, therefore, by allowing himself to be treated as the lowliest and most negligible member of society, as an outcast, had nothing further to lose and could chide even the king, making the fool in a paradoxical sense the highest and most powerful member of society. This powerless power must often have led not only to humor but to feelings of self-hate in the fool, feelings which required aggressive expression not only through ordinary jests but through extraordinary jests. Till Eulenspiegel is said to have eaten his own feces in court in order to shame the courtiers, but clearly the very act itself must have been repugnant even to Till. In a 1604 English pamphlet called *Jack of Dover's Quest of Inquiry* we find a section telling of a number of "knights," but it is significant that the section is called "The Fool of Cornwalle." In the following case history, the "fool" is a fool in name only, an outcast aggressively expressing his opinion of society:

> I was told of a humorous knight dwelling in
> the same countrey (that is, Cornwalle), who
> upon a time, having gathered together in one

> open market-place a great assemblie of
> knights, squires, gentlemen, and yeomen, and
> whilest they stood expecting to heare some
> discourse or speech to proceed from him, he,
> in a foolish manner (not without laughter),
> began to use a thousand jestures, turning his
> eyes this way and then that way, seeming
> always as though presently he would have
> begun to speake, and at last, fetching a deepe
> sigh, with a grunt like a hogge, he let a beastly
> loud fart, and tould them that the occasion of
> this calling them together was to no other end
> but that so noble a fart might be honoured
> with so noble a company as there was.

There was not only aggression in this performance but also, obviously, premeditation.

The most famous farters of history have been those who could not only express themselves through flatulence, like the tailor or the fool, but who could express themselves at length and at will. There are numerous recorded instances. The first important record of voluntary public farting is found in *The City of God* (411) by St. Augustine. Book 14, chapter 24 concerns "The power of the will over the body" and argues that one result of expulsion from the Garden of Eden was the loss of a certain degree of physical responsiveness to mental control. Augustine notes that "We do in fact find among human beings some individuals with natural abilities very different from the rest of mankind and remarkable by this very rarity." Falling into this category are "A number of people [who] produce at will such musical sounds from their behind (without any stink) that they seem to be singing from that region."

Michel de Montaigne, the great French essayist who was also a physician, takes up the question of flatulence in chapter 20 of his first book of essays. He seems almost aware of the modern theory of diverticulosis when he writes that:

> I could heartily wish that I only knew...how oft a man's belly, by the denial of one single puff, brings him to the very door of an exceeding painful death.

In this chapter, called "Of the Force of Imagination" (1580), Montaigne notes Augustine's report of singing flatulation and acknowledges Augustine's later commentator Vives' additional eye-witness account of a similar concert. Notwithstanding these instances, Montaigne remained skeptical towards noble, singing farts and considered them only a means to express aggression, if not against society then against oneself. He relates a sorry account of what must surely quality as one of history's great farters:

> I myself know one [anus] so rude and ungoverned as for forty years kept its master at work with one continued and unintermitted hurricane, and 'tis like will do so till he expire that way.

But in all fairness to the farters of the world, the greatest of them all was not by his passing of gas also passing a judgment. His completely conscious control of his abilities was confirmed by numerous chemical examinations, including two in published form. This man, a hero at bottom, was a gentle and loving father, a noble and steadfast friend, a successful and generous businessman, and a great stage entertainer. This unique individual, a phenomenon among phenomena, this explosive personality and credit to our subject, was christened Joseph Pujol, but invented for himself the name by which all history knows him: Le Petomane!

Le Petomane could fart as often and as frequently as he wished. Like the people Augustine mentions, his farts were odorless: the air he expelled from this anus had just previously been inhaled through his anus. As other people use their mouths, Le Petomane had learned to use his anus. Furthermore, by constricting or loosening his anus he could vary the pitch of the air he expelled and by controlling the force of abdominal contraction he could control its loudness. With these two fundamental tools, simple enough but rarely seen, Le Petomane contrived to imitate not only the farts of modest virgins or wild animals, but to make music. He headlined at the Moulin Rouge in Paris, the most famous nightclub in the world at that time, and brought in box office receipts more than twice as high as those of the angelic Sarah Bernhardt. He was one of the greatest comedians of the turn of the century. The manager of the Moulin Rouge kept nurses in the theater to tend to female customers whose uncontrolled laughter in tight corsets often caused them to pass out as Le Petomane passed gas. Here was not a court fool at all but the toast of civilized society. He arrived in Paris like a bombshell.

Joseph Pujol was born on the first of June, 1857, in his family's bourgeois home at 13 rue des Incurables in Marseille. Thirteen is usually thought of as a jinxing number, but Joseph's oddity, which most of us would think a liability, became his passport to immortality. Indeed, great people make their own luck. It was fortunate that this malady was not "incurable."

As a boy, Joseph had had a frightening experience in the sea. Holding his breath and ducking underwater, he suddenly felt a rush of cold water enter his bowels. He went to find his mother but was embarrassed to see water running out of himself. Although he recounted this in later years, apparently as a child he tried to keep this terrifying experience a secret. Like any well-brought-up child of his social class, Joseph remained tight-lipped and followed the life course his parents had laid out for him. He went to school until the age of thirteen, became apprenticed to a baker, and when his apprenticeship was complete he set up his own bakery in a shop built for him by his father François, a stone mason.

In 1883 he married Elizabeth Henriette Oliver and soon thereafter commenced to build a family at the rate of one child every two years for a total of ten children, all of whom he apparently doted upon and all of whom, apparently, worshipped him.

Early in his married life he was called to military service and in the boisterous, all-male atmosphere of the barracks he recounted for the first time his strange experience in the sea. Joseph was always a gentle and accommodating person and, when asked for a demonstration, he agreed to try again. On their next furlough, he and his unit went to the sea. He did succeed in taking water in and then letting it out. This might have been viewed as mere freakishness, but combined with Joseph's gentleness and good humor, this struck the soldiers as a delightful feat.

Pujol, using a basin, practiced this art in private with water and, once able to control the intake and outflow by combined exertions of his anal and abdominal muscles, he soon began to practice with air as well. This, of course, only for his own amusement and the occasional amusement of his fellow soldiers.

When he returned home he resumed his life as a baker and father but added to it his new found love of entertainment. He began to work part-time in music halls as an ordinary singer, as a trombone player, and soon as a quick-change artist with a different costume for each song. He began to add comic routines of this own writing to his singing and playing acts and was quite popular locally. At the same time he began to turn his special ability into an act, learning to give farts as imitations. Soon his friends urged him to add this to his act but he was diffident about the propriety of such a thing. Instead, in order to give it a try, he rented a theater of his own. He was an almost instant success. Still diffident, despite his love of the music halls and his growing popularity, he did not trust himself to a stage career quite yet. Instead, he left the bakery in care of his family and went to a number of provincial capitals, and at each stop Le Petomane played to packed houses. His farts drove them *in*. Finally, in 1892, he blew into Paris.

The Moulin Rouge (the Red Mill) was his aim and with his provincial success behind him, as it were, he went right for that famous club. The building was topped by a small set of windmill sails and Pujol was reputed to have said, as he first approached this landmark, "What a marvelous fan for my act." The manager of the Moulin Rouge, one Oller, on hearing of Le Petomane's specialty, was astounded at Pujol's audacity but agreed to give him an audition. In Paris as in Marseille, the act was an instant success.

Le Petomane would begin by walking out dressed quite elegantly in silks and starched white linen, a thorough swell.

69

It's a Gas

"Ladies and Gentlemen, I have the honor to present a session of Petomanie. The word Petomanie [which Pujol had first given air to] means someone who can break wind at will but don't let your nose worry you. My parents ruined themselves scenting my rectum." This combination of irony and anatomical honesty inspired his act and won over the patrons of Paris. After his opening monologue Le Petomane leaned forward, hands on knees, turned his back to the audience, and began his imitations. "This one is a little girl," he would say and emit a delicate, tiny fart. "This one is a mother-in-law," he'd say, and there would be a slide. "This is a bride on her wedding night," very demure indeed, "and this the morning after," a long, loud one. Then he would do a dressmaker tearing two yards of calico, letting out a crackling, staccato fart that lasted at least ten seconds, and then cannonfire, thunder and so on. The public loved the act and the actor; the Moulin Rouge gave him an immediate contract. In a short time, he was their headliner.

His act grew with his popularity. Among other feats he could mix in to the performance were those dependent upon inserting a rubber tube in his rectum (very decorously passed through his pocket). With this tube he could amiably chat away while at the same time smoking a cigarette. Sometimes he would insert a six-stop flute into the tube and accompany his own singing. A few simple nursery tunes he could play without recourse to the tube at all. And finally, he would almost always end his acts by blowing out a few of the gas-fired footlights. All that was left, before rising and bowing out, was to invite the audience to join him, and they did with hysterical gusto, their own convulsed abdomens insuring that many of the patrons could indeed participate in the group farting at the appropriate moment. Le Petomane's act was a liberating experience for all and he was much in demand.

The management of the Moulin Rouge kept their headliner on a tight reign — he was, after all, unique. But a few performances outside that hall were encouraged. For one thing, they wanted Le Petomane to submit to medical examination so that his authenticity would be even more accepted and this he did not only for the sake of his career but as yet another mark of his characteristic complacency. For similar reasons of believability, Oller allowed Pujol to give private performances for all-male audiences at which he could perform wearing pants with an appropriate cut-out. Before these events, and before his regular performances as well, he thoroughly washed himself by the method he had practiced in the army, sitting into a basin, drawing water in and then shooting it out. He also began every day this way for all his long life and to these unique enemas attributed his never having experienced a single day of illness. Whether that effect is so or not, it is certainly true that these washings prevented Pujol's farts from carrying any odor or flammable gases. Thus his performances public and private alike were not offensive to the nose or dangerous to the theater. In the smaller groups he would extinguish a candle at the distance of a foot and demonstrate his water jet over a range of four or five yards. These distances are also corroborated by medical observation.

The Moulin Rouge, acting as Le Petomane's agent, also encouraged him to travel abroad. As one can imagine from a knowledge of the cultures involved, he was not well received by the Arabs in northern Africa and the Spaniards insisted that he act a clown instead of a petomane. But in other European countries, and especially in Belgium, he was a star attraction. At his private performances in France, where no admission was charged, Pujol would finish by passing the hat, hand to hand that is. At one of these gatherings a man leaned forward and put a 20 louis gold piece in the hat. When Pujol, astonished, asked how much change the man wanted, he leaned forward again and told him to keep it, that the show was worth it although he had had to travel from Brussels to see it. He had heard so much about Le Petomane but could not see him in his own country because his own movements were so closely watched there. So he had come from Paris that night incognito to see and hear the great Le Petomane. He was King Leopold II of Belgium.

Pujol's stage life was not unrelievedly happy, however. Oller kept this sociable man to a very hard contact and demanded long hours from him. Despite Le Petomane's fame, Pujol never abandoned his working friends. This kindness led to a legal action which is doubtless the largest case ever hinging on a fart. One day, on his own time, Pujol visited the stall of a gingerbread lady who was not faring well. To help her business pick up a bit, and catch the attention of the public, he did a few "simple airs" in the open market. Oller, in order to demonstrate his exclusive contractual power, demanded that Pujol pay the Moulin Rouge the 3,000 franc fine stipulated in the contract for performing on his own. When Pujol refused, Oller filed suit. This finally decided Le Petomane to set up his own traveling Theater Pompadour and regain the independence he had had as a baker in Marseille. From 1894 to 1914 Pujol performed in this theater, usually in Paris but sometimes in the provinces, and for these twenty years was able to be with his family on a constant basis, always working and joking together. The Great War, which enlisted Pujol's four sons, brought the entertainment to a stop. One son became a prisoner-of-war and two others were invalided. After the Armistice, this world famous comic hadn't the heart to continue. Instead, he used his wealth to set up his children in bakeries and two in bread factories and with them he managed these and other businesses, living a long and prosperous life.

The lawsuit was one of the few things in life that went completely against Pujol. He seemed not to care about that decision though, because it was rendered in the early days of his traveling theater. Still, he was galled at Oller and galled to have to pay the money, equivalent to nearly $2,000 today, a fine just for farting for a friend. However, Pujol had his revenge. Oller, anxious not to lose his patrons to the Theater Pompadour, employed a "female petomane" named Angele Thiebeau who "farted" by means of a bellows concealed under her skirt. Pujol sued her and the Moulin Rouge for fraudulent imitation. At the same time, a reviewer, doubtless part of Le Petomane's loyal public, wrote up her act as a sham, dependent on a cheap trick lacking in skill and utterly devoid of Le Petomane's own humane charm. She and Oller sued the reviewer for slander. The wheels of justice grind exceedingly slow, but they do grind and finally the reviewer was vindicated, Oller reprimanded and Thiebeau publicly disgraced. The outcome of Pujol's own suit seemed assured, but, in a typical gesture, his point having been made, he withdrew the action.

Pujol was genuinely a good ole fart. He never forgot his family and friends nor the demands of proper society. At a fancy dinner he was once asked by the hostess, while at table, to demonstrate his skill. He glanced at this companion to the right, a Captain of Artillery, and replied simply, "When this gentleman has fired his cannon, I will speak." His fame occasioned numerous satiric songs and pamphlets, any of which might have been actionable had Pujol been contentious. But he was so widely viewed as gentle and kind that the satirists never defamed Pujol himself and he himself never took their words with anything but good humor.

The Medical Faculty at the Sorbonne offered Pujol 25,000 francs for the right to examine his body after his death. He was a vigorous man, a proud patriarch, and, knowing what such a sum could mean to his children and grandchildren, he accepted. But, despite the fact that he had distinguished himself publicly displaying himself for so many years, he was held in such regard by those around him that, on his peaceful demise in 1945 at the age of 88, the family refused the offer. And so, having made flatulence a subject not for aggression but for pleasantry, Joseph Pujol, the greatest farter in history, came to his proper end.

CHAPTER FIVE

Fart Gallery
— *a pictorial extravaganza* —

> *God, if this were enough,*
> *That I see things bare to the buff.*

Robert Louis Stevenson, 1887

Fart art is a rare commodity, as well it might be. After all, it isn't easy to draw a picture of something that can't be seen. But the effects of farts are as visible as the wrinkled noses in an elevator stuck between floors, and artists of sensitivity have captured our airy somethings with their pencils and brushes and chisels. Herewith, a small but pungent collection of minor artistic explosions.

Aubrey Beardsley (1872-1898) was an English illustrator well known for his unusual depictions of classic scenes. In this etching from 1896, *Lysistrata Defending the Acropolis*, Beardsley imagines one of the ways in which the leader of a women's sex strike in ancient Greece (described in Aristophanes' play of 412 B.C.), kept the men at bay. This is a case in which the best defense is clearly to give offense.

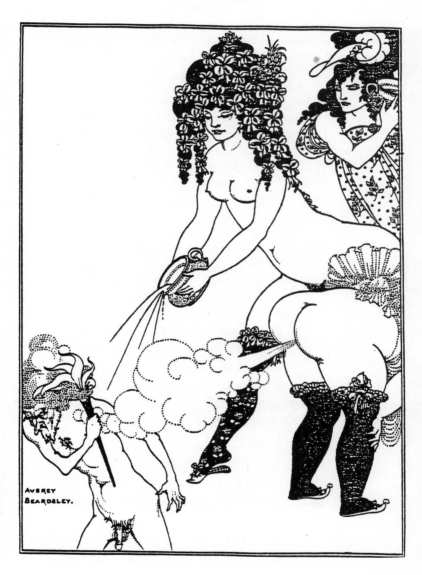

Pieter Brueghel (1520-1569) was a Dutch painter who also recognized the danger of exploding farts. In this large and famous painting depicting one hundred twenty *Flemish Proverbs* (1559) he pictures a common medieval toilet arrangement: a wooden outhouse built onto a stone building and over-hanging a river or moat. The two would-be evacuators have above them a man holding an "executioner's bill" used for public beheading. This Flemish proverb is literally "shitting below the gallows" or, in English equivalent, "sitting on the edge of a volcano." While the exposed buns seem indifferent to the nearby danger, the man in the river below them and to the right seems to have gotten wind of something rather distressing. It's a good thing he has a fan.

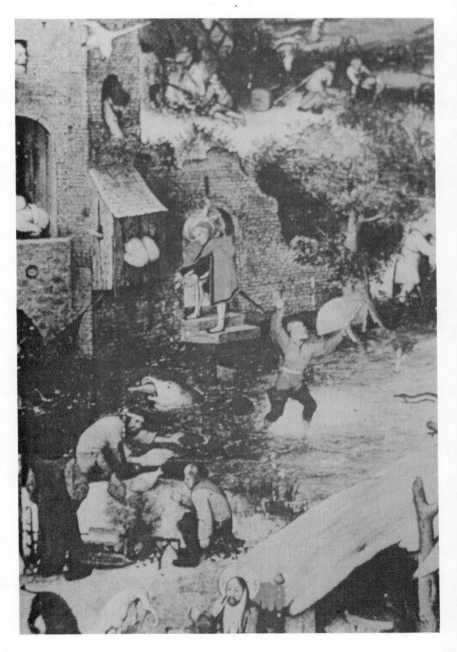

Of course, not everyone wants to avoid farts. Here we have a *fifteenth-century Belgian relief sculpture* that very well illustrates another proverb: There is no accounting for taste.

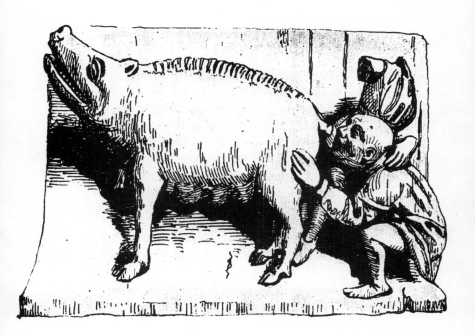

Perhaps farts would be more widely appreciated if we could turn them to good purpose. From ancient times, as this engraving of the miniature on a *Roman onyx ring* shows, people, even those with extraordinary nasal development, have tried to set the fart to music.

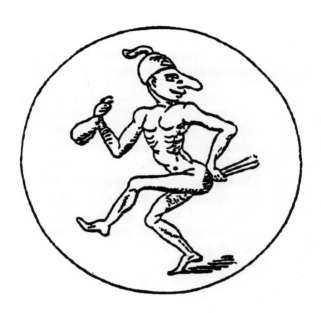

Another entertaining idea that people keep slipping out has a certain explosive appeal. Remember when you first heard about lighting farts? It seemed like a new idea. Well, like so many other things we believed in our youth, that notion, as the following *fifteenth-century Belgian relief* shows, was just so much hot air.

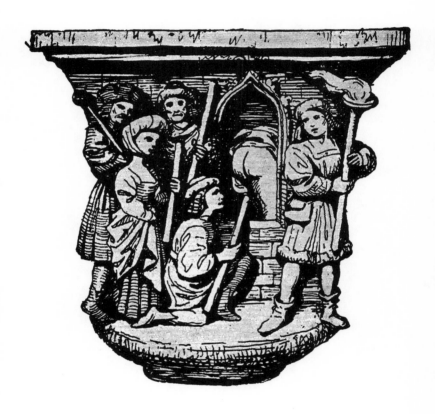

Just because an idea is old, however, doesn't mean it isn't good. After all, if one could only harness the fart one could start a new industry: natural gas. Apparently the sixteenth-century Belgians were already on to that idea — and they weren't even worried about an oil embargo.

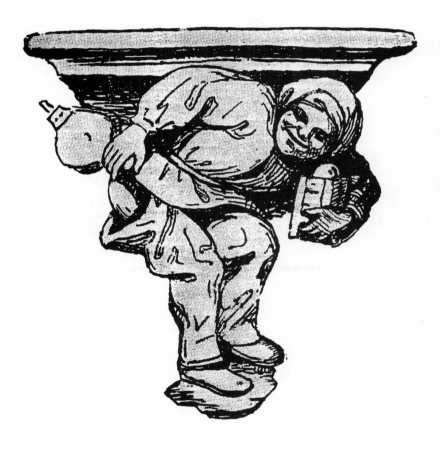

Unfortunately, as this 1801 scientific etching by **James Gillray** (1757-1815) shows, early nineteenth-century science proved conclusively that the idea of harnessing the fart for power just couldn't pass muster.

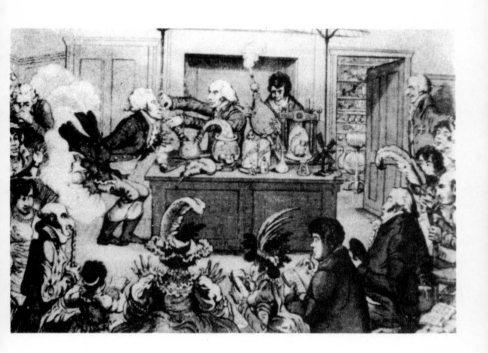

Undaunted by having thus bombed out, science turned its eyes — and noses — to the skies. Perhaps, as this 1827 etching attributed to **John Phillips** indicates, many may have gotten from the birds not only the idea of winged flight but of jet propulsion itself.

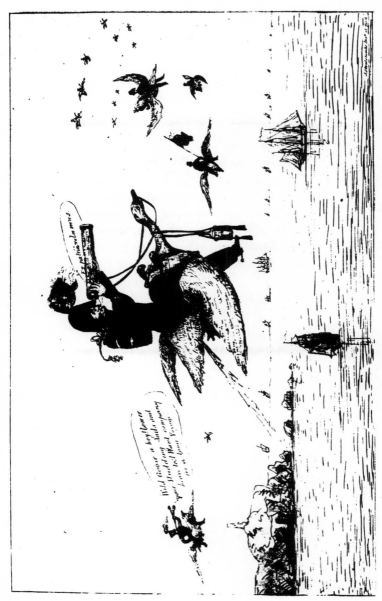

James Ensor (1860-1949) was a Belgian satiric painter who felt that the jet fart was definitely *not* for the birds, as he makes clear in his 1888 etching called *Wizards in a Squall*.

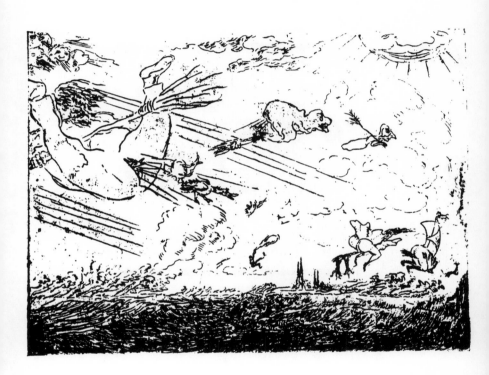

Ensor, besides producing noxious demons and foul fowl, conceived of farts as providing one-fifth of his society's *Doctrinal Nourishment* (1889). What constitutes the rest of the food of the masses is left to the reader's keen senses.

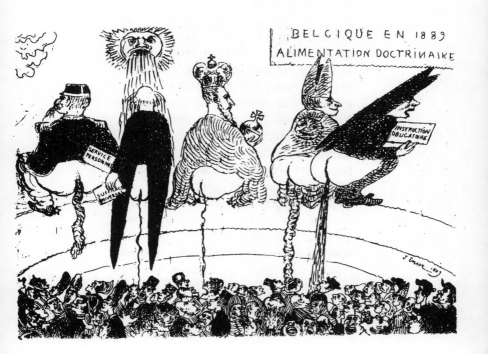

Indeed, although the fart is invisible in itself, it does occupy a place in our art and may even serve as part of a grand vision. **Hieronymus Bosch** (1450-1516) was yet another Dutchman who simply had to deal with our subject. Lest one infer from all these Belgian and Dutch fart artists that the Low Countries really are low, one should note that Bosch's great triptych, *The Garden of Earthly Delights* (1514), treats farts quite elevatedly. In this catalog of pleasures, toward the bottom of the central panel, occupying a place just below the salt-water fish — a symbol of voluptuousness — we find an age-old dream come true in oils: a portrait of someone who can actually fart roses. How sweet it is!

Fart Gallery

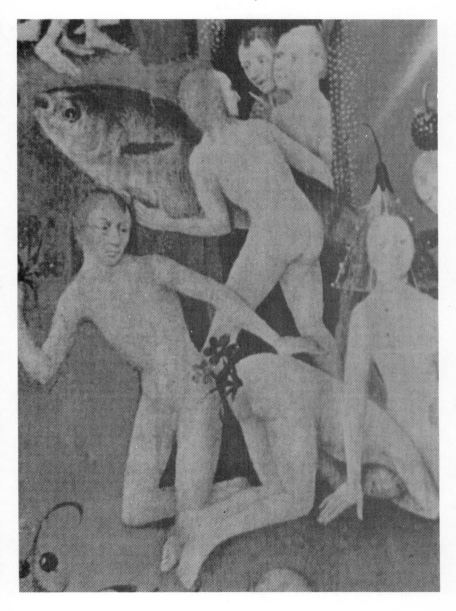

In *The Garden of Earthly De-lights*, **Bosch** not only imagined the miracle of a farter who smelled like roses but, equally miraculous, he was able to fore-see fart delights nearly four hun-dred years ahead. In this detail drawn from the right-hand panel of the great triptych, we see a poor soul both bearing his giant-sized flute as a burden and simul-taneously playing his ordinary-sized flute à la Joseph Pujol. Art knows no bounds!

Fart Gallery

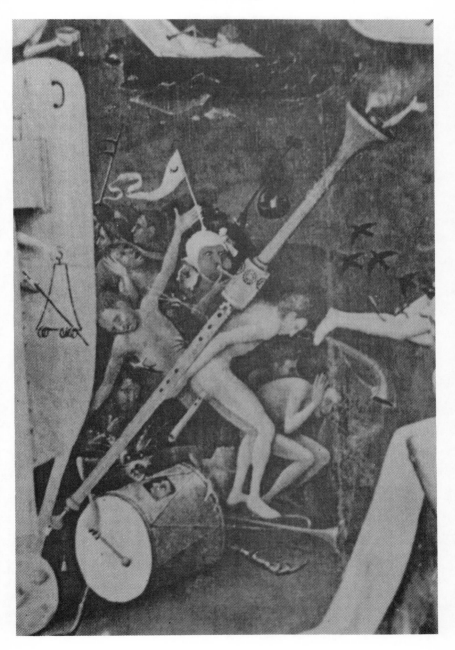

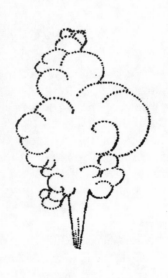

CHAPTER SIX

A Fragrant Nosegay
— a literary anthology —

My Words *are few, but spoke with* Sense.
And yet my speaking *gives Offense.*

Jonathan Swift, 1724

Just as farts have been suppressed in our society, and the discussion of farts along with them, much good literature by some of the world's great (and not so great) writers has been suppressed as well. We intend to correct that situation right now. In this chapter we present for your sensitive... eyes... some of the best fart literature there is. Sit down, hold open the covers, and have a blast!

*****

The most ancient Western humorist of whom we still have complete works is the Greek dramatist Aristophanes. In *The Clouds* (423 B.C.) he satirizes the reputedly atheistic Socrates and the Sophistic school of philosophy. Socrates and his student engage in dialogue, the latter wondering what might cause the thunder and lightning. Not Zeus, Socrates explains, but the crepitations of the clouds. The answer is blowin' in the wind.

It's a Gas

from *The Clouds*

Student: Whence then, my friend, does the thunder descend?
        that does make me quake with affright!

Socrates: Why 'tis they, I declare, as they roll through the air.

Student: What the Clouds? did I hear you aright?

Socrates: Ay: for when to the brim filled with water they swim,
        by Necessity carried along,
    They are hung up on high in the vault of the sky,
        and so by Necessity strong
    In the midst of their course, they clash with great
    force,
        and thunder away without end.

Student: But is it not He who compels this to be?
        does not Zeus this Necessity send?

Socrates: No Zeus have we there, but a Vortex of air.

Student: What! Vortex? that's something, I own.
    I knew not before, that Zeus was no more,
        but Vortex was placed on this throne!
    But I have not yet heard to what cause you referred
        the thunder's majestical roar.

Socrates: Yes, 'tis they, when on high full of water they fly,
        and then, as I told you before,
    By Compression impelled, as they clash, are compelled
        a terrible clatter to make.

A Fragrant Nosegay

Student: Come, how can that be? I really don't see.

Socrates: Yourself as my proof I will take.
      Have you never then eat the broth-puddings you get
           when the Panathenaea comes round,
      And felt with what might your bowels all night
           in turbulent tumult resound?

Student: By Apollo, 'tis true, there's a mighty to-do,
           and my belly keeps rumbling about;
      And the puddings begin to clatter within
           and kick up a wonderful rout:
      Quite gently at first, papapax, papapax,
           but soon pappapappax away,
      Till at last, I'll be bound, I can thunder as loud,
           papapappappapappax, as They.

Socrates: Shalt thou then a sound so loud and profound
           from thy belly diminutive send,
      And shall not the high and the infinite Sky
           go thundering on without end?
      For both, you will find, on an impulse of wind
           and similar causes depend.

Student: Well, but tell me from Whom comes the bolt through
           the gloom, with its awful and terrible flashes;
      And wherever it turns, some it singes and burns,
           and some it reduces to ashes!
      For this 'tis quite plain, let who will send the rain,
           that Zeus against perjurers dashes.

Socrates: And how, you old fool of a dark-ages school,
           and an antediluvian wit,
      If the perjured they strike, and not all men alike,

It's a Gas

           have they never Cleonymus hit?
    Then of Simon again, and Theorus explain:
           known perjurers, yet they escape.
    But he smites his own shrine with his arrows divine,
           and "Sunium, Attica's cape,"
    And the ancient gnarled oaks: now what prompted
           those strokes?/ *They* never forswore I should say.

Student: Can't say that they do: your words appear true.
               Whence comes then the thunderbolt, pray?

Socrates: When a wind that is dry, being lifted on high,
               is suddenly pent into these [clouds].
       It swells up their skin, like a bladder, within,
               by Necessity's changeless decrees:
       Till, compressed very tight, it bursts them outright,
               and away with an impulse so strong,
       That at last by the force and the swing of its course,
               it takes fire as it whizzes along.

Student: That's exactly the thing that I suffered one Spring,
               at the great feast of Zeus, I admit:
       I'd a paunch in the pot, but I wholly forgot
               about making the safety-valve slit.
       So it spluttered and swelled, while the saucepan I held,
               till at last with a vengeance it flew:
       Took me quite by surprise, dung-bespattered my eyes,
               and scalded my face black and blue!

                    *****

A Fragrant Nosegay

The most famous farting scene in all literature is probably the closing episode of the tale told by the pilgrim miller in *The Canterbury Tales* of Geoffrey Chaucer (d. 1400). Often omitted from expurgated editions of the classic collection, this bawdy story depicts jealousy and infidelity in the most earthy of terms. Old John the carpenter has wed himself to the most comely maiden in Oseney, eighteen-year old Alison — and he is unfailingly jealous of her. In John's household, besides the chore-boy Robin and the maid Jill, there resides an Oxford student called in the story "handy Nicholas." *Handy* has three meanings here: first, the word reminds us that Nicholas is available because he lives in the same house with the wife John wants to protect; second, Nicholas is a capable fellow, able to fix up any little household problem; and third, he has a subtle way of making his affections for Alison apparent; he sticks his hand between her legs and hangs on until she consents to spend the night with him if only he can arrange it in safety. At this point it seems that Chaucer has arranged an example of "the eternal triangle." But not so. In fact, "The Miller's Tale" is more like an infernal square, for there's another man on the scene, Absolom the parish clerk, a lecherous and foppish priest who has most of the women in the county but has especial pangs for delicious Alison. Unlike the more direct Nicholas, he makes his desires known by whispers and singing. In fact, he is as famous for his music as for his fastidiousness: "No tavern anywhere/ But he had furnished entertainment there./ Yet if a man broke wind, he winced a bit,/   And spoke with delicacy, no word unfit." Alison, however, does not respond to Absolom's sophisticated approach.

105

It's a Gas

In order to provide himself with a trysting time, Nicholas executes a bizarre scheme designed to play on John's uneducated credulity. First Nicholas stays up in his room noiselessly for days, until finally John sends Robin to see if Nicholas is ill. The amateur astrologer is found sitting upright in bed, eyes and mouth agape, apparently mad. When John himself comes up, Nicholas explains that he has divined the near approach of another Noah's flood. At John's urging, Nicholas tells what must be done. First, no one must be told of all this. Second, the servants must be sent away. Third, working in secret, John must outfit a large kneading-trough for himself, another for Alison, and another for Nicholas. Each trough should have a full day's supply of food, for the flood will come and recede again in the space of twenty-four hours. In order that the neighbors not see these preparations, the troughs should be hung up under the roof, approachable by ladder and provided with tools for cutting holes in the roof to escape when the waters rise. John does as he is told and late Sunday night all three retire to their separate troughs, vowed to silent prayer the better to obtain God's favor. The scene thus set, we can pick up the last parts of Chaucer's famous tale:

From *The Miller's Tale*

The dead of sleep, for very weariness,
Fell on this carpenter, and I should guess,
At about curfew times, or little more.
His head was twisted, and that made him snore.
His spirit groaned in its uneasiness.
Down from his ladder slipped this Nicholas,
And Alison too, downward she softly sped
And without further word they went to bed

Right where the carpenter slept on other nights.
There were the revels, there were the delights!
And so this Alison and Nicholas lay
Busy about their solace and their play
Until the bell for lauds began to ring
And in the chancel friars began to sing.
        Now on this Monday, woebegone and glum
For love, this parish clerk, this Absolom
Was with some friends at Oseney, and while there
Inquired after John the carpenter.
A member of the cloister drew him away
Out of the church, and told him, "I can't say.
I haven't seen him working hereabout
Since Saturday. The abbot sent him out
For timber, I suppose. He'll often go
And stay at the granary a day or so.
Or else he's at his own house, possibly.
I can't for certain say where he may be.
        Absolom all at once felt jolly and light,
And thought, "Time now to be awake all night,
For certainly I haven't seen him making
A stir about his door since day was breaking.
Don't call me a man if when I hear the cock
Begin to crow I don't slip up and knock
On the low window by his bedroom wall.
To Alison at last I'll pour out all
My love-pangs, for at this point I can't miss,
Whatever happens, at the least a kiss.
Some comfort, by my word, will come my way.
I've felt my mouth itch the whole livelong day,
And that's a sign of kissing at the least.
I dreamed all night that I was at a feast.
So now I'll go and sleep an hour or two,
And then I'll wake and play the whole night through."

107

It's a Gas

When the first cockcrow through the dark had come
Up rose this jolly lover Absolom
And dressed up smartly. He was not remiss
About the least point. He chewed licorice
And cardamon to smell sweet, even before
He combed his hair. Beneath his tongue he bore
A sprig of Paris like a truelove knot.
He strolled off to the carpenter's house, and got
Beneath the window. It came so near the ground
It reached his chest. Softly, with a half a sound,
He coughed, "My honeycomb, sweet Alison,
What are you doing, my sweet cinnamon?
Awake, my sweetheart and my pretty bird,
Awake, and give me from your lips a word!
Little enough you care for all my woe,
How for your love I sweat wherever I go!
No wonder I sweat and faint and cannot eat
More than a girl; as a lamb does for the teat
I pine. Yes, truly, I so long for love
I mourn as if I were a turtledove."
        Said she, "You jack-fool, get away from here!
So help me God, I won't sing 'Kiss me, dear!'
I love another more than you. Get on,
For Christ's sake, Absolom, or I'll throw a stone.
The devil with you! Go and let me sleep."
        "Ah, that true love should ever have to reap
So evil a fortune," Absolom said, "A kiss,
At least, if it can be no more than this,
Give me for love of Jesus and of me."
        "And will you go away for that?" said she.
        "Yes, truly, sweetheart," answered Absolom.
        "Get ready then, " she said, "for here I come,"
And softly said to Nicholas, "Keep still,
And in a minute you can laugh your fill."

A Fragrant Nosegay

Thus Absolom got down upon his knee
And said, "I am a lord of pure degree,
For after this, I hope, comes more to savor.
Sweetheart, your grace, and pretty bird, your favor!"
      She undid the window quickly. "That will do,"
She said. "Be quick about it, and get through,
For fear the neighbors will look out and spy."
      Absolom wiped his mouth to make it dry,
The night was pitch dark, coal-black all about.
Her rear end through the window she thrust out.
It fared no better or worse with Absolom
Than with his mouth to kiss her naked bum
Before he had caught on, a smacking kiss.
      He jumped back, thinking something was amiss.
A woman has no beard, he was well aware,
But what he felt was rough and had long hair.
      "Alas," he cried, "what have you made me do?"
      "Te-hee!" she said, and banged the window to.
Absolom backed away a sorry pace.
      "You've bearded him!" said handy Nicholas.
"God's body, this is going fair and fit!"
This luckless Absolom heard every bit,
And gnawed his mouth, so angry he became.
He said to himself, "I'll square you, all the same."

Absolom, rubbing his lips and muttering words of
revenge, goes to a blacksmith and talks him into lending him
the colter which he is at that very moment heating to work
into the front edge of a plowshare. He:

    took the colter where the steel was cold
    And slipped out with it safely in his hold
    And softly over to the carpenter's wall.
    He coughed and then he rapped the window, all

It's a Gas

As he had done before.
          "Who's knocking there?"
Said Alison.   "It is a thief, I swear."
          "No, no," said he.   "God knows, my sugarplum,
My bird, my darling, it's your Absolom.
I've brought a golden ring my mother gave me,
Fine and well cut, as I hope that God will save me.
It's yours, if you will let me have a kiss."
          Nicholas had got up to take a piss
And thought he would improve the whole affair
This clerk, before he got away from there,
Should give *his* ass a smack; and hastily
He opened the window, and thrust out quietly,
Buttocks and haunches, all the way, his bum.
Up spoke this clerk, this jolly Absolom:
"Speak, for I don't know where you are, sweetheart."
          Nicholas promptly let fly with a fart
As loud as if a clap of thunder broke,
So great he was nearly blinded by the stroke,
And ready with his hot iron to make a pass,
Absolom caught him fairly on the ass.
          Off flew the skin, a good handbreath of fat
Lay bare, the iron so scorched him where he sat.
As for the pain, he thought that he would die,
And like a madman he began to cry,
"Help! Water! Water! help, for God's own heart!"
          At this the carpenter came to with a start.
He heard a man cry "Water!" as if mad.
"It's coming now," was the first thought he had.
"It's Noah's flood, alas, God be our hope!"
He sat up with his ax and chopped the rope
And down at once the whole contraption fell.
He didn't take time out to buy or sell
Until he hit the floor in a dead swoon.

A Fragrant Nosegay

Then up jumped Nicholas and Alison
And in the street began to cry, "Help, ho!"
The neighbors all came running, high and low,
And poured into the house to see the sight.
The man still lay there, passed out cold and white,
For in his tumble he had broken an arm.
But he himself brought on his greatest harm,
For when he spoke he was at once outdone
By handy Nicholas and Alison
Who told them one and all that he was mad.
So great a fear of Noah's flood he had,
By some delusion, that in his vanity
He'd bought himself these kneading-troughs, all three,
And hung them from the roof there, up above,
And he had pleaded with them, for God's love,
To sit there in the loft for company.
        The neighbors laughed at such a fantasy,
And round the loft began to pry and poke
And turned his whole disaster to a joke.
He found it was no use to say a word.
Whatever reason he offered, no one heard.
With oaths and curses people swore him down
Until he passed for mad in the whole town.
Wit, clerk, and student all stood by each other.
They said, "It's clear the man is crazy, brother."
Everyone had his laugh about this feud.
So Alison, the carpenter's wife, got screwed
For all the jealous watching he could try,
And Absolom, he kissed her nether eye,
And Nicholas got his bottom roasted well.
God save this troop! That's all I have to tell.

*****

111

It's a Gas

François Beroalde de Verville (1558-1612) has come down to us with a reputation as one of the cleverest and most licentious satirists of all times. Unfortunately, reputation is about all one ever sees of Beroalde. His best known work, *Moyens Parvenier* (*The Means to Success*, 1610) is a collection of stories so delightful and so off-color that they have been suppressed for hundreds of years and never publicly printed in this country. We hope that by offering the following tale from the famous collection, Beroalde's achievements will henceforth be in good odor.

A Tale of Fair Imperia

... The matter that befell the Sieur de Lierne, a gentleman of France, who lay with a gay lady of Rome. She, after the manner of her chaste profession, had got on a sort of fine and dainty pellicles, filled with scented air; and thus girt about with odoriferous wind-bags, the fair Imperia listened to the gentleman's suit. In the midst of the play the lady put down her hand to one of the little bladders, and with a motion of her leg made it explode. The gentleman heard the noise, and was somewhat alarmed, but Imperia held him fast. "'Tis not what you think," said she, "a man should know before he fears." At this he put down his head and smelt a pleasant and delectable odour, not at all like what he had expected. After several trials he asked whether these sweet gales were wafted from her shores, as his experiences with the ladies of his native land had not prepared him for the flavour. She answered this with a philosophic frisk, and some remarks on the balmy airs of Italy and its aromatic delicacies, at which the French gentleman was greatly astonished. However, after several of these musk-shots, there came an explosion of nature and not art, and on the gentleman's putting down his head, he found himself the victim of misplaced confidence. "Alas!" quoth he, "what is this?" "'Tis a piece of courtesy," quoth she, "to put you in mind of your native land."

*****

Jonathan Swift (1667-1745) is best known as the author of *Gulliver's Travels* (1726), a delightful satire that contains, among other scenes of heroism, the fearless Gulliver saving the Palace of the minute Lilliputians from a devastating fire: he stands over the conflagration of the doll-sized structure and pees the fire out. It is surprising that while *Gulliver's Travels* is considered a classic children's tale, the following poem, no less delicate in subject and treatment, had to be retrieved in our century from the obscurity of manuscript. "The Problem" (1699) is to decide who has actually been the lover of the Regent. It seems his Lordship lets fly with gaseous as well as liquid emissions at the most passionate moments. To curry favor, then, the ladies won't stay in waiting but try to arouse their windy friend, blow for blow. A careful reading as of lines 41-42, will, we *suspect*, reveal much that is at first hidden by perfumed phrases.

It's a Gas

The Problem

Did ever Problem thus perplex,
Or more employ the Female Sex?
So sweet a Passion who cou'd think
Jove ever form'd to make a Stink?
The Ladys vow, and swear they'll try,
Whether it be a Truth, or Lye.
Love's Fire, it seems, like inward Heat,
Works in my Lord by Stool and Sweat,
Which brings a Stink from ev'ry Pore,
And from behind and from before;
Yet, what is wonderful to tell it,
None but the Fav'rite Nymph can smell it.
　　　But now, to solve the Nat'ral Cause
By sober, Philosophick Laws,
Whether all Passions, when in Ferment,
Work out, as Anger does in Vermin?
So, when a Weasel you torment,
You find his Passion by his Scent.
We read of Kings, who in a Fright,
Tho' on a Throne, wou'd fall to white.
Beside all this, deep Scholars know,
That the main String of Cupid's Bow,
Once on a Time, was an Asses Gut,
Now to a nobler Office put,
By Favour, or Desert preferr'd
From giving Passage to a Turd.
But still, tho's fixt among the Stars,
Does sympathize with Human Arse.
Thus when you feel an hard-bound Breech
Conclude Love's Bow-String at full Stretch;
Till the kind Looseness comes, and then
Conclude the Bow relax'd again.

A Fragrant Nosegay

And now the Ladys all are bent,
To try the great Experiment;
Ambitious of a Regent's Heart
Spread all their Charms to catch a Fart;
Watching the first unsav'ry Wind,
Some ply before, and some behind.
My Lord, on Fire amidst the Dames,
Farts like a Laurel in the Flames.
The Fair approach the speaking Part,
To try the Back-way to his Heart;
For, as when we a Gun discharge,
Altho' the Bore be ne'er so large,
Before the Flame from Muzzle burst.
Just at the Breech it flashes first:
So from my Lord his Passion broke,
He farted first, and then he spoke.
The Ladys vanish, in the Smother,
To confer Notes with one another;
And now they all agree, to name
Whom each one thought the happy Dame:
Quoth Neal, whate'er the rest may think,
I'm sure 'twas I that smelt the Stink.
You smell the Stink? by God you lye,
Quoth Ross, for, I'll be sworn, 'twas I.
Ladys, quoth Levens, pray forbear,
Let's not fall out; We all had Share.
And, by the most we can discover,
My Lord's an universal Lover.

*****

Another Swift satire well worth our perusal is "The Wonderful Wonder of Wonders" (1712). We reprint it with the original footnotes and postscript which, though apparently the work of an editor, were in fact written by Swift himself. This piece purports to describe an individual, but actually concerns something quite different. Since, as it says in the postscript to the piece, "it is well known, that it has been the policy of all times, to deliver down important subjects by emblem and riddle," we will not say precisely what that something is. However, it does provide a fitting context for the subject of this book.

The Wonderful Wonder of Wonders

There is a certain person lately arrived at this city, of whom it is very proper the world should be informed. His character may perhaps be thought very inconsistent, improbable, and unnatural; however, I intend to draw it with the utmost regard to the truth. This I am the better qualified to do, because he is a sort of dependant upon our family, and almost of the same age; though I cannot directly say I have ever seen him. He is a native of this country, and has lived long among us; but, what appears wonderful, and hardly credible, was never seen before, by any mortal.

It is true, indeed, he always chooses the lowest place in company; and contrives it so, to keep out of sight. It is reported, however, that in his younger days he was frequently exposed to view, but always against his will, and was sure to smart for it.

As to his family, he came into the world a younger brother, being of six children the fourth in order of birth;* of which the eldest is now head of the house; the second and third carry arms; but the two youngest are only footmen: some indeed add, that he has likewise a twin brother, who lives over against him, and keeps a victualling house⁺; he has the reputation to be a close, gripping, squeezing fellow; and that when his bags are full, he is often needy; yet when the fit takes him, as far as he gets he lets it fly.

When in office, no one discharges himself, or does his business better. He has sometimes strained hard for an honest livelihood; and never got a bit, till everybody else had done.

One practice appears very blamable in him; that every morning he privately frequents unclean houses, where any modest person would blush to be seen. And although this be generally known, yet the world, as censorious as it is, has been so kind to overlook this infirmity in him. To deal impartially, it must be granted that he is too great a lover of himself and very often consults his own ease, at the expense of his best friends: but this is one of his blind sides; and the best of men I fear are not without them.

---

*He alludes to the manner of our birth, the head and arms appear before the posteriors and the two feet, which he calls the footman. [Original].

⁺The belly, which receives and digests our nourishment. [Original].

He has been constituted by the higher powers in the station of receiver general, in which employment some have censured him for playing fast and loose. He is likewise overseer of the golden mines, which he daily inspects, when his health will permit him.

He was long bred under a master of arts,# who instilled good principles into him, but these were soon corrupted. I know not whether this deserves mention; that he is so very capricious, and to take it for an equal affront, to talk either of kissing or kicking him, which has occasioned a thousand quarrels: however, nobody was ever so great a sufferer for faults, which he neither was, nor possibly could be guilty of.

In his religion he has thus much of the quaker, that he stands always covered, even in the presence of the king; in most other points a perfect idolater,** although he endeavors to conceal it; for he is known to offer daily sacrifices to certain subterraneous nymphs, whom he worships in a humble posture, prone on this face, and stript stark naked; and so leaves his offerings behind him, which the priests++ of those goddesses are careful

---

#Perius: *magister artis, ingeniique largitor venter.* [Original].

**Alludes to the sacrifices offered by the Romans to the Goddess Cloacina. [Original].

++Gold-finders, who perform their office in the nighttime; but our author farther seems to have an eye to the custom of the heathen priests stealing the offerings in the night; of which

enough to remove, upon certain seasons, with the utmost privacy at midnight, and from thence maintain themselves and families. In all urgent necessities and pressures, he applies himself to these deities, and sometimes even in the streets and highways, from an opinion that those powers have an influence in all places, although their peculiar residence be in caverns under ground. Upon these occasions, the fairest ladies will not refuse to lend their hands to assist him: for, although they are ashamed to have him seen in their company, or even so much as to hear him named; yet it is well known, that he is one of their constant followers.

In politics, he always submits to what is uppermost; but he peruses pamphlets on both sides with great impartiality, though seldom till every body else has done with them.

His learning is of a mixed kind, and he may properly be called a *helluo librorum*, or another Jacobus de Voragine; though his studies are chiefly confined to schoolmen, commentators, and German divines, together with modern poetry and critics: and he is an atomic philosopher, strongly maintaining a void in nature, which he seems to have fairly proved by many experiments.

I shall now proceed to describe some peculiar qualities, which, in several instances, seem to distinguish this person from the common race of other mortals.

His grandfather was a member of the rump parliament, as the grandson is of the present, where he often rises, sometimes grumbles, but never speaks. However, he lets nothing pass willingly, but what is well digested. His

---

see more in the story of Bel and the Dragon. [Original].

courage is indisputable, for he will take the boldest man alive by the nose.

He is generally the first abed in the family, and the last up; which is to be lamented; because when he happens to rise before the rest, it has been thought to forbode some good fortune to his supervisors.

As wisdom is acquired by age, so, by every new wrinkle## in his face, he is reported to gain some new knowledge.

In him we may observe the true effects and consequences of tyranny in a state: for, as he is a great oppressor of all below him, so there is nobody more oppressed by those above him; yet in his time, he has been so highly in favour, that many illustrious persons have been entirely indebted to him for their preferments.

He has discovered, from his own experience, the true point wherein all human actions, projects, and designs do chiefly terminate; and how mean and sordid they are at the bottom.

It behooves the public to keep him quiet; for his frequent murmurs are a certain sign of intestine tumults.

No philosopher ever lamented more the luxury, for which these nations are so justly taxed; it has been known to cost him tears of blood;*** for in his own nature he is far from being profuse; though indeed he never stays

---

##This refers to a proverb--you have one wrinkle in your a-se more than you had before. [Original].

***Hemorrhoids, according to the physicians, are a frequent consequence of intemperance. [Original].

a night at a gentleman's house, without leaving something behind him.

He receives with great submission whatever his patrons think fit to give him; and when they lay heavy burdens upon him, which is frequently enough, he gets rid of them as soon as he can; but not without some labour, and much grumbling.

He is a perpetual hanger on; yet nobody knows how to be without him. He patiently suffers himself to be kept under, but loves to be well used, and in that case will sacrifice his vitals to give you ease; and he has hardly one acquaintance, for whom he has not been bound; yet, as far as we can find, was never known to lose anything by it.

He is observed to be very unquiet in the company of a Frenchman in new clothes, or a young coquette.[+++]

He is, in short, the subject of much mirth and raillery, which he seems to take well enough; though it has not been observed, that ever any good thing came from himself.

There is so general an opinion of his justice, that sometimes very hard cases are left to his decision: and while he sits upon them, he carries himself exactly even between both sides, except where some knotty point arises, and then he is observed to lean a little to the right or left, as the matter inclines him; but his reasons for it are so manifest and convincing, that every man approves them.

[+++]Their tails being generally observed to be most restless. [Original].

It's a Gas

Postscript

Gentle Reader,

Though I am not insensible how many thousand persons have been, and still are, with great dexterity handling this subject, and no less aware of what infinite reams of paper have been laid out upon it; however, in my opinion, no man living has touched it with greater nicety, and more delicate turns, than our author. But, because there is some intended obscurity in this relation; and curiosity, inquisitive of secrets, may possibly not enter into the bottom and depth of the subject, it was thought not improper to take off the veil, and gain the reader's favour by enlarging his insight. *Ars enim non habet inimicum, nisi ignorantem.* It is well known, that it has been the policy of all times, to deliver down important subjects by emblem and riddle, and not to suffer the knowledge of truth to be derived to us in plain and simple terms, which are generally as soon forgotten as conceived. For this reason, the heathen religion is mostly couched under mythology. For the like reason (this being a FUNDAMENTAL in its kind) the author has thought fit to wrap up his treasure in clean linen, which it is our business to lay open, and set in a due light; for I have observed, upon any accidental discovery, the least glimpse has given a great diversion to the eager spectator, as many ladies could testify, were it proper, or the case would admit.

The politest companies have vouchsafed to smile at the bare name; and some people of fashion have been so little scrupulous of bringing it in play, that it was the usual saying of a knight, and a man of good breeding, that whenever he rose, his a-se rose with him.

*****

While Western writers broke new literary ground by breaking wind, the fabulists of the fabulous Orient were not to be left behind — as it were. Perhaps the most famous collection of Oriental literature is that which usually goes under the name of *The Thousand and One Arabian Nights*. First introduced to Europe by a French translation of 1704-1717 and into English by a translation from the French beginning in 1706, these marvelous tales immediately took hold of the Western imagination. Everyone came to know of Sinbad and Aladdin and various fascinating genies. But it wasn't until 1882-1884 that a complete translation of all thousand and one tales was made from Arabic into English. In this veritable library of fantasy, and especially at the height of the era of Queen Victoria, it is little wonder that a little tale like the following might pass unnoticed. Doubtless Abu Hasan wished he had the same luck.

The Historical Fart

It is related that in the town of Kaukaban, in Yemen, there was once a bedouin of the Fadhli tribe called Abu Hasan, who, having given up the life of the desert and settled down as a townsman, became, after much diligence and enterprise, a merchant of considerable wealth.

His wife had died while they were both young, and his friends were always pressing him to marry again. Weary of the widower's life, he at length gave in to their persuasions and engaged the services of an experienced marriage-broker, who found him a bride as beautiful as the moon when it shines on the sea. He celebrated the wedding with a sumptuous feast, to which he invited his near and distant kinsfolk, the ulema and fakirs of the town, and friends and acquaintances from all over the countryside. His whole house was thrown open to the wedding guests. There was rice of every hue and flavour, sherbets, lambs stuffed with walnuts, almonds, and pistachios, and a young camel roasted whole. Everyone ate, drank, and made merry; and the bride was displayed, according to custom, in seven different robes — and again in yet another robe as befitted such a grand occasion — to the great joy of the women, who marvelled at her exceptional beauty.

At last came the moment when Abu Hasan was summoned to the bridal chamber. Slowly and solemnly he rose from this divan; but, horror of horrors, being bloated with meat and drink, he let go a long and re-sounding fart. The embarrassed guests, whose attentions had been fixed upon the bridegroom, turned to one another speaking with raised voices and pretending to have heard nothing at all. Abu Hasan was so mortified with shame that he wished the ground would open up and swallow him. He mumbled a feeble excuse, and, instead of going to the bridal chamber, went straight to the courtyard, saddled his horse, and rode off into the night, weeping bitterly.

After a long journey he reached Lahej, where he boarded a ship ready to sail for India, and in due course arrived in Calicut on the Malabar Coast. Here he met many Arabs, especially from Hadramaut, and was recommended by them to the King, who, though an unbeliever, took him into his service and in time promoted him to the captainship of his bodyguard.

He lived there in peace and contentment for ten years, and at the end of that time he was seized with a longing for his native land as strong as that of a lover pining for his loved one, so that he almost died of his self-imposed exile.

One day, unable to resist this yearning any longer, he absconded from the King's palace, boarded a ship, and eventually landed at Makalla in Hadramaut. Here he disguised himself in the rags of a dervish and, keeping his name and identity secret, travelled to Kaukaban on foot, enduring hunger, thirst and exhaustion, and braving a thousand dangers from lions, snakes, and ghouls. By and by he reached the hill which overlooked his native town. He gazed upon his old house with tears in his eyes, saying to himself: 'Pray God, no one will ever recognize me. I will first wander about the town and listen to the people's gossip. Allah grant that after all these years no one will remember what I did.'

He went round the outskirts of the town, and, as he sat down to rest at the door of a hut, he heard the voice of a young girl within, saying: 'Please mother, what day was I born on? One of my friends wants to tell my fortune.'

'My daughter,' replied the woman solemnly, 'you were born on the very night of Abu Hasan's fart.'

When he heard these words, he got up and fled. 'Abu Hasan,' he said to himself, 'the day of your fart has become a date which will surely be remembered till the end of time.'

It's a Gas

He travelled on until he was back in India, where he remained in exile until his death. May Allah have mercy upon him.

*****

Benjamin Franklin (1706-1790) was well known to have tried his hand at everything: printer, publisher, postmaster, inventor, writer and sage. It was not only his hand that he tried, however. This randy devil was so active during his years as American envoy to France that it has been asserted Franklin is ancestor to a sizable fraction of the current population of the country. (And they call George Washington "father of his country"!) In his lifetime, Franklin saw many of his public-minded suggestions taken up and brought to good effect, including the establishment of a public post office and the organization of civic security forces. The following project is in the form of a letter to the Royal Academy of Brussels. We believe it highly appropriate that Franklin addressed his suggestion to this particular body. First, the subject itself always comes up after the eating of Brussels sprouts; and second, Franklin himself — and this is important for a full understanding of the project — was a vegetarian. Franklin's suggestions often became reality, as with the creation of the first corps for public sanitation and the first public library. Unfortunately, the combination of these seems to have worked against publication of the following satire and it had to be retrieved from manuscript in this century.

A Fragrant Nosegay

To the Royal Academy of Brussels

Gentlemen:

I have perused your late mathematical prize question, proposed in lieu of one in natural philosophy for the ensuing year.... I conclude therefore that you have given this question instead of a philosophical, or, as the learned express it, a *physical* one, because you could not at the time think of a physical one that promised greater *utility*.... Permit me then humbly to propose one of that sort for your consideration, and through you, if you approve it, for the serious inquiry of learned physicians, chemists, etc., of this enlightened age.

It is universally well known that, in digesting our common food, there is created or produced in the bowels of human creatures a great quantity of wind.

That the permitting this air to escape and mix with the atmosphere is usually offensive to the company, from the fetid smell that accompanies it.

That all well-bred people, therefore, to avoid giving such offense, forcibly restrain the efforts of nature to discharge that wind.

That so retained contrary to nature it not only gives frequently great present pain, but occasions future diseases such as habitual cholics, ruptures, tympanies, etc., often destructive of the constitution and sometimes of life itself.

Were it not for the odiously offensive smell accompanying such escapes, polite people would probably be under no more restraint in discharging such wind in company than they are in spitting or in blowing their noses.

My prize question therefore should be: To discover some drug, wholesome and not disagreeable, to be mixed with our common food, or sauces, that shall render the natural discharges of wind from our bodies not only inoffensive, but agreeable as perfumes.

That this is not a chimerical project and altogether impossible, may appear from these considerations. That we already have some knowledge of means capable of *varying* that smell. He that dines on stale flesh, especially with much attention of onions, shall be able to afford a stink that no company can tolerate; while he that has lived for some time on vegetables only, shall have that breath so pure as to be insensible to the most delicate noses; and if he can manage so as to avoid the report, he may anywhere give vent to his griefs, unnoticed. But as there are many of whom an entire vegetable diet would be inconvenient, and as a little quicklime of fetid air arising from the vast mass of putrid matter contained in such places, and render it rather pleasing to the smell, who knows but that a little powder of lime (or some other thing equivalent), taken in our food, or perhaps a glass of limewater drunk at dinner, may have the same effect on the air produced in and issuing from our bowels? This is worth the experiment. Certain it is also that we have the power of changing by slight means the smell of another discharge, that of our water. A few stems of asparagus eaten shall give our urine a disagreeable odor; and a pill of turpentine no bigger than a pea shall bestow on it the pleasing smell of violet. And why should it be thought more impossible in nature to find means of making perfume of our wind than of our water?

For the encouragement of this inquiry (from the immortal honor to be reasonably expected by the inventor), let it be considered of how small importance to mankind, or to how small a part of mankind have been useful those discoveries in science that have heretofore made philosophers famous. Are there twenty men in Europe, this day the happier, or even the easier, for any knowledge they have picked out of Aristotle? What comfort can the vortices of Descartes give to a man who has whirlwind in his bowels! The knowledge of Newton's mutual *attraction* of the particles of matter, can it afford ease to him who is racked by their mutual *repulsion*, and the cruel distentions it occasions? The pleasure arising to a few philosophers, from seeing, a few times in their lives, the threads of light untwisted, and separated by a Newtonian prism into seven colors, can it be compared with the ease and comfort every man living might feel seven times a day, by discharging freely the wind from his bowels? Especially if it be converted into a perfume; for the pleasures of one sense being little inferior to those of another, instead of pleasing the *sight*, he might delight the *smell* of those about him, and make numbers happy, which to a benevolent mind must afford infinite satisfaction. The generous soul, who now endeavors to find out whether the friends he entertains like best claret or Burgundy, champagne or Madeira, would then inquire also whether they chose musk or lily, rose or bergamot, and provide accordingly. And surely such a liberty of *expressing one's scentiments*, and pleasing one another, is of infinitely more importance to human happiness than that liberty of the *press,* or of *abusing one another,* which the English are so ready to fight and die for.

In short, this invention, if completed, would be as Bacon expresses it, *bringing philosophy home to men's business and bosoms.* And I cannot but conclude that in comparison therewith for *universal* and *continual utility,* the science of the philosophers above-mentioned, even with the addition, gentlemen, of your *'figure quelconque,'* and the figures inscribed in it, are all together, scarcely worth a

Fart-hing

*****

The humor of Mark Twain (1835-1910) really needs little more introduction than the mention of *Tom Sawyer* (1876), *Huckleberry Finn* (1884), and *A Connecticut Yankee in King Arthur's Court* (1889). Like the last of these, the piece that follows is set in the past, but is quite different in subject matter from the better known works. For that reason, despite its excellent comedy, "1601" was suppressed for a quarter century after its composition in the 1870s. It will be easier to read this piece if one remembers that both "and" and "an" sometimes mean "if" or "and if" in the language of the times of Queen Elizabeth I and "ye," being just a typesetter's abbreviation for "the," should be pronounced like the modern word "the." Those who would relish more of "1601" than we have provided will, we trust, be able to sniff it out for themselves.

A Fragrant Nosegay

From *1601*

"1601" or conversation as it was at the fireside in the time of the tudors

(MEM: — The following is supposed to be an extract from the diary of the Pepys of that day, the same being cupbearer to Queen Elizabeth. It is supposed that he is of noble and ancient lineage; that he despises these canaille; that his soul consumes with wrath to see the queen stooping to talk to such; and that the old man feels his nobility defiled by contact with Shakespeare, etc., and yet he has got to stay there till Her Majesty chooses to dismiss him.)

Yesternight took her Majesty, ye Queene, a fantasie such as she sometimes hath, and hadde to her closet certain that do write playes, bookes & such like — these being my Lord Bacon, his worship, Sir Walter Raleigh, Mr. Ben Jonson, & ye childe Francis Beaumont, which being but sixteen hath yet turned his hand to ye doing of the Latin masters into our English tongue with great discretion and much applause. Also came with those ye famous Shaxpur. A right strange mingling of mightie bloode with meane, ye more in especial since ye Queene's Grace was present, as likewise these following, to wit: Ye Duchess of Bilgewater, twenty-two years of age; Ye countess of Granby, thirty-six; her doter, ye Lady Helen; as also ye two maides of honor, to wit: Ye Lady Margery Bothby, sixty-five; ye Lady Alice Dillbury, turned seventy, she being two yeares ye Queene's Grace's elder.

It's a Gas

I, being Her Majestie's cup bearer, hadde no choice but to remain & behold rank forgot, & ye high hold converse with ye low as upon equal termes, & a great scandal did ye world heare thereof.

In ye heate of ye talke, it befel that one did breake wynde, yielding an exceeding mightie and distressful stinke, whereat all did laffe full sore, and then:

YE QUEENE: Verily, in mine eight and sixty yeares have I not heard the fellow of this blast. Me seemeth by ye greate sound and clamour of it, it was male, yet ye bellie it did lurke behinde should now falle lene and flat against ye spine of him that hath been delivered of so stately & so vaste a bulke, whereas ye guts of them that doe quiff-spliters beare, stand comely, still & rounde. Prithee, let ye author confess ye offspring. Will my Lady Alice testify?

LADY ALICE: Goode, your Grace, an' I hade roome for such a thundergust within mine ancient bowels, 'tis not in reason I could discharge the same and live to thank God for that he did chuse handmayd so humble to show his power. Nay, 'tis not I that have brought forth this rich o'ermastering fog, this fragrant gloom, so pray seek ye further.

YE QUEENE: Mayhap ye Lady Margery hath done ye companye this favour?

LADY MARGERY: So please you, Madame, my limbs are feeble with ye weight and drouthe of five and sixty winters, & it behooveth that I be tender with them.

132

A Fragrant Nosegay

In ye goode providence of God, an' hadde I contained this wonder forsooth would I have given ye whole evening of my sinking life to ye dribbling of it forthe with trembling and uneasy soul, not launched it sudden in its matchless might, taking my own life with violence, rending my weak frame like rotten rags. It was not I, your Majestie.

YE QUEENE: In God's name who hath favoured us? Hath it come to pass that a wynde shall break itself? Not such a one as this I trow. Young Master Beaumont? But no, twould have wafted him to Heaven like downe of goose's bodie. 'Twas not ye little Lady Hellen, — nay, ne'er blush my child, thou'lt tickle thy tender mouth with many a mousie squeak before thou learn'st to blow a hurricane. Was't you, my learned and ingenious Jonson?

JONSON: So felle, a blast hath ne'er mine ears saluted, nor yet a stenche so all-pervading & immortal. 'Twas not a novice did it, good Your Majestie, but one of veteran experience — else had he failed of confidence. In sooth it was not I.

YE QUEENE: My Lord Bacon?

LORD BACON: Not from my lene entrails hath this prodigie burst forth, so please Your Grace. Nau't doth so befit ye greate as greate performance; and haply shall ye find that 'tis not from mediocrity this miracle hath issued.

133

(Though ye subject be but foul wynde, yet will this tedious sink of learning ponderously philosophize. Meantime did ye foul and deadly stinke pervade all places to that degree, that never smelt I ye like, yet dared I not leave ye Presence, albeit I was like to suffocate.)

YE QUEENE: What saith your worshipful Master Shaxpur?

SHAXPUR: In ye greate hands of God, I stande course of nature, yet hadde I not believed it; but hadde said, "ye Pit itself hath furnished forth ye stinke and Heaven's artillery hath shook ye globe in admiration of it."

(Then there was silence, & each did turne him toward ye worshipful Sir Walter Raleigh, that browned, embattled bloudy swash-buckler, who rousing up did smile and simpering say:)

RALEIGH: Most Gracious Majestie. 'Twas I that did it; but, indeed, it was so poor and fragile a note compared with such as I am wont to furnish, that in sooth I was ashamed to call ye weakling mine in so august a Presence. It was nothing — less than nothing — Madame. I did it but to clear my nether throat; but hadde I come prepared then hadde I delivered something worthie. Beare with me, please your Grace, till I can make amends.

(Then delivered he himself of such a godless and rock-shivering blaste, that all were fain to stop their ears, and following it did come so dense and foul a stinke, that that which went before did seem a poor and triffling thing beside it. Then said he, feigning that he blushed and was confused, "I perceive that I am weake today & cannot justice doe unto my powers," and sat him down as who should say, — "There, it is not much; yet he that hath the power to spare, let him follow that, an' I think he can." By God, and I were ye Queene, I would e'en tip this swaggering braggard out o' ye court & let him air his grandeurs and break his intolerable wynd before ye deaf & such as suffocation pleaseth.)

Then fell they to talk about ye manners and customs of many peoples...

Then conversed they of religion & the mightie works of ye olde dead Luther did doe by ye grace of God. Then next about poetry, & Master Shaxpur did read a part of his King Henry IV, the which it seemed unto mee is not of the value of so much ashes, yet they praised it bravely, one and all.

The same did rede a portion of his Venus & Adonis to their prodigious admiration, whereas I, being sleepy & fatigued withal, did deeme it but paltry stuffe & was ye more discomfitted in that ye bloudy buccanneer hadde got wynde again & did turn his mind to breaking wynde with such villain zeal that presently I was like to choke once more. God damn this wyndy ruffian & all his breede. I would that helle might get him...

*****

135

It's a Gas

Émile Zola (1840-1902) is the best known novelist in the tradition called "naturalism." This aesthetic ideology calls for the minute recording of things as they are, getting in every little detail, mentioning every wart on the body politic. Because such depiction often revealed the causes of social ills, indeed sometimes brought these ills to public attention for the first time, Zola's work was widely admired not only as an artistic accomplishment but as a political one as well. In *La Terre* (*The Earth*, 1887), Zola turned his attention to the peasantry and, keeping to form, recorded every little detail. In the passage that follows, we have the interactions of a fellow named Jésus-Christ (with no religious significance intended), his father Old Fouan, his daughter La Trouille, and a bailiff named Vimeux. Unfortunately for Zola's reputation, these peasants, though admittedly brutalized by the upper classes, were shown to be quite unrefined in their own right, a circumstance that Zola's liberal backers did not find sweet. Zola not only suggested just how foul these people might be, but he had the bad grace to join in the peasant's own zest and treat it all as funny.

From *La Terre*

Jésus-Christ was a very windy fellow. Continual explosions blew through the house and livened things up. Damn it all, no one could ever be bored in that rascal's house, for he never let fly without blurting out some joke or other as well. He despised timid little squeaks, smothered between the cheeks, squirting out uneasily and ashamedly. He never emitted anything but frank detonation, substantial and ample as cannon-shots. Whenever he raised his leg and settled himself with a comfortable and tactical motion, he called his daughter in tones of urgent command, with a grave expression on his face:

'La Trouille, hurry, for God's sake!'

She rushed up and the blast went off point blank with such a vibrating energy that she gave a jump.

'Run after it. Get hold of it between your teeth and see if there's any knots in it!'

At other times, as soon as she reached him he would give her his hand. 'Pull hard, draggle-tail! Make it go off with a bang!'

Then when the explosion occurred with the roar and splurge of a tightly-jammed charge, 'Ah, that was a hard one, thanks all the same.'

At other times again, he raised an imaginary gun to his shoulder and took a long and careful sight; then after the shot was fired, he shouted, 'Find it out now, retrieve it, you lazy bitch!'

La Trouille choked and fell over on her backside with laughter. The joke never palled; in fact it was funnier every time. It made no difference that she knew the game inside-out and awaited the thunderous blast that was to round it off, he always transported her with the vivid comedy of his rowdy act. O, what a joker she had for a father! Sometimes he talked of a lodger who never paid his rent and whom he had to throw out; sometimes he turned round with a grimace of surprise and bowed gravely as if the table had bidden him good morning; sometimes he had a whole posy of explosions, one for M. le Curé, one for le Maire, and another for the ladies. The fellow's belly, you'd have almost thought was a musical box from which he could extract any sound he liked; so much so that in the *Jolly Ploughman* at Cloyes they used to bet him: 'It's one on me if you let off six'; and he discharged six broadsides and won an overwhelming victory. He had gained quite a name with his knack and La Trouille was extremely proud of it. As soon as he stuck out his behind, she began laughing and wriggling in anticipation; and she was unflagging in her admiration for his prowess, gripped by the mingled fear and affection he inspired in her.

On the very evening when Old Fouan moved into the Château, as people called the old cellar where the poacher had buried himself, at the very first meal served by the girl, who stood behind her father and grandfather like a respectful servant, the jollifications were launched with loud eruptions. The old man had contributed five francs; and a tempting smell rose from the kidney-beans and the veal and onions which the young girl was an adept at cooking in a mouth-watering way. As she brought in the beans she almost dropped the dish in her fits of helpless laughter. Jésus-Christ, before sitting down, let off three regular reports, full-blast.

'Gun-salute for the feast! Now we can set to.'

Then, bracing himself, he achieved a fourth, unique, tremendous and insulting.

'That's for those rotten Buteaus. Hope it'll choke them!'

Old Fouan, who had been very downcast since his arrival, let out a sudden chuckle. He nodded his head in approval. The ceremony put him at his ease, for he too had been famous in his time as a joker. In his house the children had been brought up to ignore the paternal bombardment going on all round. He leaned his elbows on the table and allowed a wave of relaxation to engulf him as he sat opposite that tall rascal of a Jésus-Christ who gazed at him with moist eyes and an air of childlike scoundrelly joviality.

'By God, Dad, we're going to put up our feet and enjoy ourselves! You'll see my scheme. Trust me, I'll pull you up out of the bog. When you're eating dust along with the moles, how will you be any better off for having denied yourself a tit-bit up here?'

A Fragrant Nosegay

Uprooted from his life-long sobriety, and craving for forgetfulness, Old Fouan found himself replying, 'Aye, it's better to stuff everything into yourself than leave a scrap for others. Your health, my boy!'

La Trouille brought on the veal and onions. There was a moment's silence. Jésus-Christ, not wanting to let the conversation languish, let out a prolonged blast which went through the straw of his chair with the whining modulations of a human cry. He immediately turned to his daughter and solemnly enquired, 'What was that you said?'

She couldn't answer, she had to sit down and hold her sides. But what finished her off, after the veal and cheese, was the final relaxation of father and son when they began smoking and drinking the brandy set out on the table. Their mouths were sticky and their brains fuddled; all attempts at talking had ended.

Slowly Jésus-Christ tilted to one side, thundered, then looked at the door and shouted, 'Come in!'

Old Fouan took up the challenge. He had been feeling out of things for some time now. He regained something of his youth, lifted his buttock, and thundered in turn, replying, 'Here I come!'

The two men slapped each other's hands, slobbering and laughing cheek to cheek. They were enjoying themselves. The scene was altogether too magnificent for La Trouille, who had collapsed on the floor. So shaken was she with wild screams of laughter that she too let off an explosion — but a tiny one, soft and musical, like the thin note of a fife in comparison with the deep organ-notes of the two men.

Indignant and disgusted, Jésus-Christ rose and extended his arm in a gesture of tragic authority.

139

It's a Gas

'Out of here, you filthy sow! Out of here, you stinkpot! By God, I'll teach you to show respect for your father and grandfather.'

He had never allowed her such a familiarity. The sport was reserved for grown-ups. He waved his hand in the air, pretending to be asphyxiated by the little flute-puff — his own, he said, only smelt of gunpowder. Then, as the culprit, very red in the face and agitated at her lapse, denied the act and struggled against dismissal he ejected her with a single shove.

'You dirty lump, go out and shake your skirt! And don't return for an hour, not till you've been properly aired.'

.....

On one point, however, father and son were fully agreed, and that was in hatred of Vimeux the bailiff, a shabby little fellow who was given the duties which his colleague at Cloyes shrank from carrying out and who ventured to visit the Château with a formal notification of judgment. Vimeux was a fag-end of a man, extremely dirty: a red nose and a pair of bleary eyes peeping out of a tangle of yellow whiskers. He was always dressed like a gentleman, with top hat, frock-coat and black trousers; but each item of clothing was badly worn and stained. He was famous in the canton for the terrible beating-up he got from the peasants whenever he came out on his own to present writs or the like against them in some area remote from aid. Tales were widely told of sticks snapped across his shoulders, dunkings in cow-ponds, a two-mile race with a pitch-fork held at his back to stimulate speed, by a mother and daughter after they'd pulled his trousers down.

When Vimeux called, Jésus-Christ was coming in with his gun; Old Fouan, smoking his pipe as he sat on a tree-trunk, growled to his son, 'See the disgrace you're bringing on our heads, you rogue!'

'Wait till you see!' the poacher muttered between his teeth.

Vimeux, noticing him and his gun, stopped some thirty paces off; the whole of his lamentable, black, dirty and correctly-attired person quaked with fear.

'Monsieur Jésus-Christ,' he said in a small shrill voice, 'I am here on the matter you know about. I'll put this down there. Good evening.'

He planted the official document on a stone and was rapidly retreating when the other shouted out.

'You damned ink-pisser, do you want me to teach you manners? Just you have the politeness to bring me that paper.'

And as the miserable creature stood rooted to the ground, terrified out of his wits and not daring to move forward or backwards, he took aim at him.

'I'll send you a bit of lead if you don't hurry. Come on, pick up your paper and bring it over here. Nearer, nearer, still nearer, you bloody coward, or I'll fire!'

Frozen pale with terror, the bailiff tottered on his short legs. He looked imploringly at Fouan. But the old man went on calmly smoking his pipe, withdrawn in his vehement hatred of the legal charges and the man who personified them in the eyes of the peasantry.

'Ah, there we are at last, it's not so bad. Give me your paper. No, not with the tips of your fingers as if you didn't want to part with it. Politely, for God's sake, and show some good will. There! that's the proper way, thanks.'

Vimeux, paralyzed by the mockery of the towering scoundrel, blinked as he awaited the threatening joke, the punch or blow which he felt sure was coming.

'Now you can turn round.'

He understood, refused to move, tensed his buttocks.

'Turn round, or I'll come and turn you myself.'

Vimeux saw that he'd have to submit. He turned sadly round and presented to view his poor little bottom as thin as a starving cat's. The poacher sprang forward vigorously and planted the toe of his boot just in the right spot with such force that the little man went flat on his face fully four yards away. He rose painfully to his feet and bolted in abject terror as he heard a further shout.

'Look out, I'm going to fire!'

Jésus-Christ's gun was at his shoulder. But he contented himself with raising his leg — and bang! He released a blurt with such a resounding crack that Vimeux, terrified at the detonation, once again fell flat. This time his black hat fell off and rolled away among the stones. He ran after it, snatched it up, then went dodging off faster than before. Behind him the shots continued — and bang! bang! bang! without a pause: a perfect fusillade accompanied by shots of laughter which completed his bewilderment. Bounding down the slope like a grasshopper, he was already a hundred yards distant, but Jésus-Christ's cannonade still echoed through the valley. Indeed the whole countryside reverberated and there was one last formidable blast as the bailiff, who from the distance now looked about the size of an ant, disappeared into Rognes. La Trouille, who had run out at the uproar, lay on the ground holding her stomach and clucking like a hen. Old Fouan had taken his pipe from his mouth so as to laugh more heartily. Ah, that devil of a Jésus-Christ, was a good-for-nothing, and yet what a funny chap when he liked.

*****

142

A Fragrant Nosegay

In an English song first published in 1855, the heroine Kathusalem is the daughter of the "Baba of Jerusalem," presumably the chief rabbi. She has the ill luck to fall in love with an infidel and the lovers meet death at her father's hands. This sad song with a nonetheless rousing melody became a beer hall favorite. In the course of not a very long time, and certainly by the end of Word War I, most versions of "Kathusalem" had left murder far behind to concentrate on other (ob)noxious matters. The particular version we present here was created by mingling a number of these later airs.

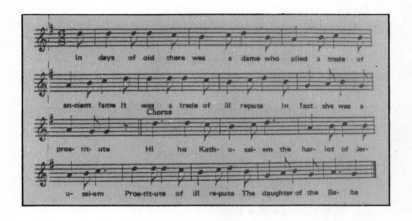

In days of old there was a dame who plied a trade of an-cient fame It was a trade of ill repute In fact she was a pros- tit- ute Hi ho Kath- u- sal- em the har- lot of Jer- u- sal-em Pros-tit-ute of ill re-pute The daughter of the Ba- ba

It's a Gas

Olde Beerhall Songs & Airs

In days of old there was a dame
Who plied a trade of ancient fame.
It was a trade of ill repute;
In fact, she was a prostitute.

Chorus:
Hi, ho Kathusalem,
The harlot of Jerusalem,
Prostitute of ill repute,
The daughter of the Baba.

And when the army came to town,
The price went up and she went down.
Her fertile field was nicely sown,
This harlot of Jerusalem.

Sadly though there was a hitch:
Kathusalem was a gassy bitch
Who maketh every nose to twitch
That liveth in Jerusalem.

There was a prince both lean and tall
Whose member was the ruin of all
Maidens who lined the Wailing Wall
That standeth in Jerusalem.

One night returning from a spree,
His customary hard had he
And on the street he chanced to meet
This harlot of Jerusalem.

A Fragrant Nosegay

He laid her down upon the grass,
Lifted her dress above her ass;
But during the act he passed some gas
While doing it to Kathusalem.

Kathusalem was over-gassed.
She arched her back and loosed a blast
That sent him flying far and fast,
Sailing o'er Jerusalem.

And when the moon is bright and red
A flying form sails overhead,
Still raining curses on the head
Of that farting whore Kathusalem.

*****

In addition to the fart literature found flying from the feckless fingers of the famous, the common can concatenate as well. And so, in order to guarantee that we have created a literary atmosphere permeated by every possible perfume from the nosegay of fartdom, we add here those verses writ by someone, but by no one known. These are the wisdom of the ages.

Traditional Verses

A belch is but a breath of air
That cometh from the heart.
But when it takes the downward path
It then becomes a fart.

It's a Gas

Here I sit, broken hearted:
Paid a nickel to shit and only farted!

Bean, beans, the musical fruit:
The more you eat, the more you toot!
The more you toot the better your feel,
So eat beans at every meal!

Of all popular verse in English, the most popular of all is surely the limerick. This venerable poetic form is found in "Sumer is icumen in," dating from about 1300, the very oldest popular song of which we have a record in our language. We present that song below in a literal modern translation using the same subjects. Note that the word "starts" means "jumps," as in the word, "startle"; the word "blows" means "blossoms"; and, most important please note that the lines we have set in italics form the first example of the only verse form exclusively native to English, the limerick:

Lilting Limericks

Summer is a'comin' in,
Loudly sing cuckcow!
The seed grows and meadow blows,
And the woods spring forth now.
Sing cuckcow!

Ewe bleats after her lamb,
After calf lows the cow.
Bullock starts,
Buck he farts,
Merry sing cuckcow!

146

A Fragrant Nosegay

Cuckcow, cuckcow,
Well you sing cuckcow:
Nor ease your nerve now!

The more modern examples of the limerick are almost invariably bawdy and many of the best bear the unmistakable odor of our subject. We are simply bursting to present them for you now. Sing cuckcow!

There was a young lady named Ames
Who would play at the jolliest games.
    She was great fun to lay
    For her rectum would play
Obbligatos, and call you bad names.

Sir Reginald Barrington, Bart.
Went to the masked ball as a fart.
    He had painted his face
    Like a more private place
And his voice made the dowagers start.

There was an old Bey of Calcutta
Who greased up his asshole with butter.
    Instead of the roar
    Which came there before,
Came a soft, oleaginous mutter.

There was a young fellow named Charted
Who rubbed soap on his bung when it smarted,
    And to his surprise
    He received a grand prize,
For the bubbles he blew when he farted.

It's a Gas

There was a young girl of La Plata
Who was widely renowned as a farter.
    Her deafening reports
    At the Argentine sports
Made her much in demand as a starter.

    A keen-scented dean of Tacoma
    Was awarded a special diploma
        For his telling apart
        Of a masculine fart
    From a similar female aroma.

The Farter From Sparta

There was a young fellow from Sparta,
A really magnificent farter,
    On the strength of one bean
    He'd fart God Save the Queen,
And Beethoven's Moonlight Sonata.

He could vary, with proper persuasion,
His fart to suit any occasion
    He could fart like a flute
    Like a lark, like a lute,
This highly fartistic Caucasian.

This sparkling young farter from Sparta,
His fart for no money would barter.
    He could roar from his rear
    Any scene from Shakespeare,
Or Gilbert and Sullivan's Mikado.

148

A Fragrant Nosegay

He'd fart a gavotte for a starter,
And fizzle a fine serenata.
  He could play on his anus
  The Coriolanus:
Oof, boom, er-tum, tootle, yum tah-dah!

He was great in the Christmas Cantata,
He could double-stop fart the Toccata,
  He'd boom from his ass
  Bach's B-Minor Mass,
And in counterpoint, La Traviata.

Spurred on by a very high wager
With an envious German named Bager,
  He'd proceed to fart
  The complete oboe part
Of a Haydn Octet in B-Major.

His repertoire ranged from classics to jazz,
He achieved new effects with bubbles of gas.
  With a good dose of salts
  He could whistle a waltz
Or swing it in razzamatazz.

His basso profundo with timbre so rare
He rendered quite often, with power to spare.
  But his great work of art,
  His fortissimo fart,
He saved for the Marche Militaire.

It's a Gas

One day he was dared to perform
The William Tell Overture Storm,
    But naught could dishearten
    Our spirited Spartan,
For his fart was in wonderful form.

It went off in capital style,
And he farted it through with a smile,
    Then, feeling quite jolly,
    He tried the finale,
Blowing double-stopped farts all the while.

The selection was tough, I admit,
But it did not dismay him one bit,
    Then, with ass thrown aloft
    He suddenly coughed..
And collapsed in a shower of shit.

His bunghole was blown back to Sparta,
Where they buried the rest of our farter,
    With a gravestone of turds
    Inscribed with the words:
"To the Fine Art of Farting, A Martyr."

And, in a somewhat more somber vein, this anonymous epigram first published in 1735:

If death must come, as oft as breath departs,
Then he must often die, who often farts;
And if to die be but to lose one's breath,
Then death's a fart; and so a fart for death.

CHAPTER SEVEN

Turning Down the Gas
— what you can do —

You don't need a weatherman to know which way the wind blows.

Bob Dylan

Just as you may not need a weatherman to know which way the wind blows, you may not need a physician to cut down on the wind's blowing. Somewhere between ten and twenty percent of all Americans are afflicted with what they themselves think of as gas excessive to the point of both pain and embarrassment. If you — or someone close, perhaps too close, to you — suffer from excessive gas, help may be within your grasp. If nothing that follows in this chapter deflates you, though, see a doctor.

There are three routes you can take to capping your gas problem: selecting foods with care, preparing them with care, and supplementing your diet. Virtually all people can mitigate their music by following one or more of these routes. First, let us consider food selection.

As mentioned in our first chapter, the most common cause of severe and painful excessive gas is a condition known as "lactose intolerance" or "lactase deficiency." Lactase is an enzyme — a chemical normally produced by the body itself — that is crucial to the digestion of so-called milk sugar, otherwise known as lactose. Lactose is ingested in milk or milk goods. In a healthy individual, the body's own lactase helps break down the lactose and the resulting small sugars are readily absorbed and used by the body. In those with a lactase deficiency, the lactose passes undigested into the large intestine where bacteria break it down through fermentation. Just as fermented beer has bubbles, so will the contents of one's large intestine. We know those bubbles as "gas."

A physician can administer a "lactose tolerance test" for you with comparative ease, but you can even more easily test your tolerance to milk and milk products simply by banning them from your diet for a couple of days, fasting for about six hours, then drinking a glass of milk, and fasting for six more hours. If you get gas, it is from the milk and you probably have a lactase deficiency. There is, of course, a foolproof cure for gas caused by lactase deficiency: stop ingesting lactose. For those for whom milk is an essential source of calcium, this untasty choice may also be dangerous, but calcium supplements and happier friends may make the trade-off worthwhile.

For most people, most flatus is simply the result of consuming foods containing substances we cannot digest ourselves but that our colonic bacteria can digest. Most of these are the famous gas-making vegetables, each of which has one form or another of complex sugars known as oligosaccharides, the main recognized source of flatus. You can test yourself by noting which of these you tend to eat, eliminating them temporarily, and then seeing what happens when you reintroduce them into your diet. Different people — depending on their individual abilities to manufacture enzymes and their individual collections of colonic bacteria — will react more or less strongly to items in the following four lists:

Légumes:

Adzuki beans
Alfalfa
Black-eyed peas
Black mung beans
Broadbeans
Chickpeas/garbanzo beans
Common beans
Cow peas
Field beans
Garden peas
Green beans
Green mung beans
Horse gram
Lentils
Lima beans
Lupins
Mung beans
Navy beans
Peanuts
Pigeonpeas
Pole beans
Red kidney beans
Split peas
Soybeans
Soyflour
Winged beans

Nuts and seeds:

Cottonseed flour
Pistachios
Sesame flour
Sunflower flour

Grains and cereals:

Amaranth
Barley
Corn
Millet/proso
Oat bran
Oat flour
Rice bran
Rye
Sorghum grain
Wheat bran
White wheat flour
Whole wheat flour

Fruits and Vegetables:

Apples
Apricots
Beets
Brussels sprouts
Cabbage
Carrots
Cauliflower

154

Chicory
Citrus fruits (oranges and so on)
Cucumber
Eggplant
Green pepper
Leeks
Lettuce
Onions
Parsley
Parsnips
Plums
Prunes
Pumpkin
Raisins
Red pepper
Salsify
Spinach
Squash

In eliminating listed items from your diet, be careful to eliminate them *entirely*. For example, if you think you may be reacting gassily to wheat, make sure you avoid bread, cake, pastries made with wheat, wheat germ, breakfast cereals containing wheat, and so on. If you think you may be reacting gassily to citrus fruits, make sure you avoid them not only whole and fresh but in jams, jellies, and candies. Once you do identify one or more culprits, of course, the simplest cure for the gas works is to avoid the culprits entirely.

For those who have not noticed a pattern connecting their diet to their gas, the most drastic but certain course is an elimination diet. On such a diet one begins by cutting down to only a small handful of foods, say coffee and celery. After a day, one reintroduces one food at each meal to one's diet, thereby determining which are culprits and which are not. Obviously, if you normally consume a wide variety of foods, learning with certainty which are fine and which are not can require a great deal of time and discipline. But for those in bad odor, an elimination diet may just eliminate their problem. But rather than simply avoiding these foods forever, one might consider better ways of preparing them.

The most frequently named gassifiers are beans. All dried beans, with the exception of lentils, need to be soaked before they are cooked. As most vegetarians know, if you discard the soak water and cook in fresh water, you cut down drastically the beans' gaseous powers. (It is also true, of course, that with the soak water go many of the water soluble vitamins such as vitamin C. Those concerned might consider whether or not to replenish these in a non-gaseous way, such as taking a daily vitamin supplement.) Indeed, most vegetables, if boiled, will experience some breakdown in their complex sugars and other complex carbohydrates, with the result that you will have done physically what the colonic bacteria were hoping to do chemically. By robbing them of their chance to ferment, you cut down your own flatus. So, for beans, throw out the soak water; for beans and all vegetables, consider boiling.

There are also biological processes that accomplish this desired breakdown of oligosaccharides. Germination of beans to sprouts, for example, robs the beans of much of their gassy power. Similarly, the fermentation of soy beans in the process of making tofu renders soy beans ungassy without losing any of the soy beans' healthful proteins. In the same way, the fermentation of milk — into yogurt, yakult, kefir, acidophilus milk, or bulgarican milk (all available in most health food

156

stores and most available in large supermarkets) — breaks down some of the lactose that so many find a problem. Look for the words "live culture" or "active culture" on these products to be sure that the benefits of biology were not thwarted by early heat treatments (pasteurization).

If, after all this, you still simply must have a food that you know is gassy for you and can't find a way to prepare it that pleases both your taste and your friends, then you might consider supplementing your diet. The candidates here are simethicone, activated charcoal, lactase, and alpha-galactosidase.

Simethicone is the most popular of the pharmacological foaming agents. It can be found in over-the-counter antacids. Simethicone works to make lots of microscopic bubbles join into a few large bubbles. Many people often have a "bloaty" feeling right after a big meal, and wish they could just burp. Simethicone helps them do just that. Unfortunately for gas sufferers, however, simethicone works only in the stomach, far upstream from the land of colonic fermentation, and does nothing to prevent flatus. But if stomach gas is your problem, you might try it.

Activated charcoal, on the other hand, does reduce flatus. Taken in sufficient quantities (usually four capsules just before a meal and four just after), this material will absorb much of the gas produced in the large intestine. Unfortunately, continued use of activated charcoal has a number of drawbacks. First, it colors one's stool black, and thus often scares people, especially those who know that a black stool is typically a sign not of eating activated charcoal but of intestinal bleeding. Second, it absorbs not only gas but other items as well, and some of these may be medicines (such as birth control pills). Even if you take no medicines, you should know that activated charcoal can absorb some vitamins and minerals essential to one's diet. Third, activated charcoal is expensive. As of this writing, the Charcocaps brand typically costs about a dollar a meal. But for those who want to be able to sneak in the capsules in private both before and after the meal, activated charcoal may be the additive of choice.

For most people, a more practical solution is to supply enzymes to the offending foods themselves before those foods enter the body. Two related companies, Lactaid, Inc. and AkPharma, Inc. make products for milk and for vegetable products respectively.

In drop form, Lactaid^R can be added to milk twenty-four hours in advance of its consumption and the consumer will then find up to ninety percent of the lactose predigested. Those who don't think ahead, or who want to consume other milk products such as cheese or ice cream, often find that chewing one or more Lactaid tables — or Natural Brands' "milk digestant tablets" — at the beginning and again in the middle of the meal, does the trick.

For the vegetable offenders, the answer is another product, sold only by AkPharma, and known as Beano^{TM}. This is available only in drop form and must be put onto the first bite of the offending food. Beano contains the enzyme alpha-galactosidase which does for most oligosaccharides what lactase does for lactose. Since the alpha-galactosidase is destroyed by heat, you must let that first forkful of beans cool somewhat before adding your few drops, but once done, the aftereffects of the meal become decidedly more pleasurable. We ran a controlled, fasting study using twenty of our gamer — and perhaps gamier — friends, and found that both according to self-report and the reports of spouses, Beano diminished the volume of flatus by nearly one-half. This confirms the figures from prior and more extensive studies. For reasons we have not been able to determine, in our small study the beneficial effect was even more pronounced for men (nearly 80% gas reduction) than for women, but given the wide variability among individuals of both genders, this fact should not dissuade anyone interested from trying Beano. A few people (especially those with known allergies to fungi) may show an allergic reaction and should then, of course, cease using the product, but for the majority who will find it innocuous, compared to activated charcoal, Beano is the clear winner: it takes nothing essential out of your body, it seems to have no frightening side effects, and it costs about twelve cents per serving of vegetables.

Given the ever more widely accepted health benefits of a low fat, low meat, high vegetable, high fiber diet, gas is likely to be an ever more pressing issue in our society. But by eating selectively, preparing food wisely, supplementing our diets... and by learning to laugh at the inevitable, we can all be glad we passed this way together.

Bon appétit!

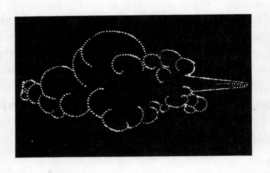

Selected Bibliography

General:

Bach, George R. and Herb Goldberg, *Creative Aggression.* New York: Avon, 1976.

Blackman, W.S. *The Fellahin of the Upper Egypt.* London: George G. Harrap & Company, Ltd., 1927.

Bourke, John G. *Scatologic Rites of All Nations.* Washington, D.C.: Lowdermilk, 1891.

Dubois, Abbe J.A. *Hindu Manners, Customs and Ceremonies.* Oxford: Clarendon Press, 1906.

Firth, Raymond, *We, the Tikopia.* London: George Allen & Unwin, Ltd., 1936.

Freud, Sigmund. "Character and Anal Erotism," 1908 in *The Standard Edition of the Complete Psychological Works of Sigmund Freud.* James Strachey, ed. London: Hogarth Press, 1957, Vol. IX.

Hartogs, Renatus. *Four-Letter Word Games.* New York: M. Evans, 1967.

Human Relations Area Files. New Haven, Connecticut: HRAF, Inc., 1974.

Hyman, Dick. *It's Still the Law.* New York: David McKay, 1961.

Junod, H.A. *The Life of a South African Tribe.* London: Macmillan & Co., 1927.

Kemp, P. *Healing Ritual.* London: Faber & Faber, Ltd., 1935.

Khaing, M.M. *Burmese Family.* Bombay: Longmans, Green & Co., 1946.

Lee, Jae Num. *Swift and Scatological Satire*. Albuquerque: University of New Mexico Press, 1971.

Legman, G. (ed.). *The Limerick*. New York: Bell, 1969.

Malinowski, Bronislaw. *The Sexual Life of Savages in North Western Melanesia*. New York: Horace Liveright, 1929.

Messing, Simon D. *The Highland Plateau Amhara of Ethiopia*. P.D. dissertation, University of Pennsylvania, 1957.

Montagu, Ashley. *The Anatomy of Swearing*. New York: Macmillan, 1967.

Nimuendaju, C. *The Eastern Timbira*. Berkeley and Los Angeles: The University of California Press, 1946.

Nohain, Jean and F. Caradec. *Le Petomane*. Los Angeles: Sherbourne Press, 1967.

Opler, M.E. *An Apache Life-Way*. Chicago: The University of Chicago Press, 1941.

Partridge, Eric. *A Dictionary of Slang and Unconventional English*. Seventh Edition. New York: Macmillan, 1970.

Rattray, R.S. *Ashanti Law and Constitution*. Oxford: Clarendon Press, 1929.

Medical:

Alvarez, W.C. "What Causes Flatulence?" *JAMA* 120:21, 1942.

Bardet, *Bull et mém de la soc de med et de chir prat de Paris*, pp. 122-124, 1894.

Davenport, H.W. *Physiology of the Digestive Tract*. 2nd Edition. Chicago: Year Book Medical Publishers, 1966.

Dougherty, R.W. "Eructations in Ruminants," *Ann. N.Y. Acad. Sci.* 150:22, 1968.

Selected Bibliography

Grosberg, S.J. "The Diagnostic Significance of Intestinal Gas," *J. Am. Geriatr. Soc.* 17:400, 1969.

Gemer, M. and Feuchtwanger, M.M. "Pneumatic Rupture of the Colon," *JAMA* 233:355, 1975.

Hussey, J.L and Pois, A.J. "Bowel Gas Explosion," *Amer. J. Surg.* 120:103, 1970.

Hickey, C.A., Calloway, D.H., and Murphy, E.L. "Intestinal Gas Production Following Ingestion of Fruits and Fruit Juices," *Am. J. Digest Dis.* 17:383, 1972.

Lasser, R.B., Bond, J.H. and Levitt, M.D. "The Role of Intestinal Gas in Functional Abdominal Pain." *N. Engl. J. Med.* 239: 524, 1975.

Levitt, M.D. "Methane Production in the Gut," *N. Engl. J. Med.* 291:528, 1974.

Levitt, M.D. "Intestinal Gas," *Postgraduate Med.* 57:77, 1975.

Levitt, M.D. "A Rational Approach to Intestinal Gas," *Viewpoints in Digest. Dis.* 9(2), March 1977.

Magendie, F. *Mémoire sur la deglutation de l'air atmospherique (1813)* quoted in Kantor, J.L. "A Study of Atmospheric Air in the Upper Digestive Tract," *Am. J. Med. Sci.* 155:829, 1918.

Machella, T.E., Dworkin, M.J., and Biel, F.T. "Observations on the Splenic Flexure Syndrome." *Ann. Int. Med.* 37:543, 1952.

Murphy, E.L., and Calloway, D.M. "The Effect of Antibiotic Drugs on the Volume and Composition of Intestinal Gas from Beans," *Digestive Diseases*, 17:639, 1972.

Price, K.R., et al. Review Article. "Flatulence--Causes, relation to diet and remedies." Die Nahrung 32:609, 1988.

Ragins, H., Shinya, H., and Wolf, W.I. "The Explosive Potential of Colonic Gas During Colonoscopic Electrosurgical Polypectomy," *Surg. Gynecol. Obstet.* 138: 554, 1974.

Roth, J.L.A. "The Symptom Patterns of Gaseousness," *Ann. N.Y. Acad. Sci.*, 150:109, 1968.

Steggerda, F.R. "Gastrointestinal Gas Following Food Consumption," *Ann. N.Y. Acac. Sci.*, 150;57, 1968.

Taylor, C.B., and Robinson, F.J. "Flatulence at Altitude in Presence of Cardiospasm," *J. Aviat. Med.* 16:272, 1945.

Wynne-Jones, G. "Flatus Retention is the Major Factor in Diverticular Disease," *Lancet*, 2:211, 1975.

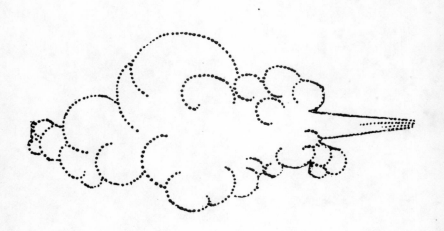